EMT-Basic®
Second Edition

EMT-Basic®

Richard J. Lapierre, M.A.
EMT-Cardiac Director
Brown University Medical Services

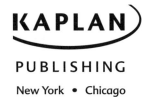

PUBLISHING

New York • Chicago

Executive Editor: Jennifer Farthing
Editors: Caryn Yilmaz and Monica Lugo
Production Editor: Samantha Raue
Production Artist: Virginia Byrne
Cover Designer: Carly Schnur

Published by Kaplan Publishing, a division of Kaplan, Inc.
888 Seventh Ave.
New York, NY 10106

Printed in the United States of America

February 2007
07 08 09   10 9 8 7 6 5 4 3 2 1

ISBN-13: 978-1-4195-5095-9
ISBN-10:   1-4195-5095-0

Library of Congress Control Number: 2005211276

Kaplan Publishing books are available at special quantity discounts to use for sales promotions, employee premiums, or educational purposes. Please call our Special Sales Department to order or for more information at 800-621-9621, ext. 4444, e-mail kaplanpubsales@kaplan.com, or write to Kaplan Publishing, 30 South Wacker Drive, Suite 2500, Chicago, IL 60606-7481.

Contents

Section III: Full-Length Practice Test and Explanations

Section IV: EMT-Basic Resources

About the Author

Rick Lapierre is the Director of Emergency Medical Services for Brown University in Providence, Rhode Island. He is a licensed Emergency Medical Technician Cardiac and a Rhode Island EMS Instructor/Coordinator. He is a retired Deputy Fire Chief from the Oakland-Mapleville Fire Department in Burrillville, Rhode Island, where he was responsible for EMS. He received a Bachelor of Science degree from the University of Rhode Island and a Master of Arts degree from Providence College. He served on the Legislative Committee that drafted the current Emergency Medical Service legislation for the State of Rhode Island and was active for many years with the Emergency Medical Services section of the International Association of Fire Chiefs. He is also Director of Emergency Management for the town of Burrillville, Rhode Island. He is married to Mary Lou Lapierre and is the father of two daughters and the proud grandfather of two granddaughters.

The author wishes to thank the following people:

There are so many people who shaped and formed me into a good EMT. My grandfather Jack Mandeville was a deputy fire chief, my father Rene Lapierre was a fire captain, and I am indebted to them for instilling in me a love of public safety and service.

Throughout my career, I learned from so many people: Chiefs like Smokey Potter, Otis Wyatt, and Mike Cosetta; EMTs and Paramedics like Gerry McVeigh, Ed Marsland, Jack Holland, Ron Gilchrist, Annie Gjelsvik, and Chris Harwood; Medical professionals like Dr. Ted Wheeler, Dr. Francis Sullivan, and Sue Connell, RN. The many Paramedics, EMTs, firefighters, and police officers I continue to work with who inspire me and make me so proud of what we all do. Who I am today and what I do as a medical professional has a small part of each one of these people, as well as hundreds of others, for we are all truly a brotherhood and a sisterhood of healers.

None of what I have accomplished, including the writing of this book, could have been done without the love and support of my wife, friend, and soul mate. She is always there when I return from a call that has been less than successful and always provides just the right word at the right time to urge me forward. None of us lives in a vacuum, nor do we really do anything by ourselves. Therefore it is with great devotion and love that I dedicate this work to my wife, Mary Lou, who in no small part is really the medical provider who has made the biggest difference in my life.

kaptest.com/publishing

The material in this book is up-to-date at the time of publication. However, the National Registry of Emergency Medical Technicians may have instituted changes in the test after this book was published. Be sure to carefully read the materials you receive when you register for the test.

If there are any important late-breaking developments—or any changes or corrections to the Kaplan test preparation materials in this book—we will post that information online at **kaptest.com/publishing.** Check to see if there is any information posted there regarding this book.

kaplansurveys.com/books

We'd like to hear your comments and suggestions about this book. We invite you to fill out our online survey form at **kaplansurveys.com/books**. Your feedback is extremely helpful as we continue to develop high-quality resources to meet your needs.

How to Use This Book

This book provides you with everything you need to ace the EMT-Basic exam. We've included this section with some tips on how to make sure you make the most of your prep time.

STEP ONE: FAMILIARIZE YOURSELF WITH THE EMT-BASIC

The first chapter of this book, Inside the EMT-Basic Exam, covers the basics of the test: what's on it, who it's for, and how to register. Once you get a sense of what's on the test, you will be ready to get a sense of yourself as a test taker. The first chapter also gives you Kaplan's exclusive test-taking strategies in a nutshell. Read this chapter carefully to learn Kaplan's proven methods for increasing your score on this challenging exam.

STEP TWO: DO THE REVIEW

Go through the content chapters paying especial attention to any weak areas. Use the bulleted lists at the beginning of each chapter to find out exactly what is in that chapter. Make sure to do the Practice Sets at the end of each chapter. Read the explanations carefully to reinforce the material, especially those for any question you got wrong.

STEP THREE: CONCLUDE YOUR PREPARATION WITH THE PRACTICE TEST

Your preparation with this book should conclude with the simulated full-length EMT-Basic exam. After completing this exam, work through the explanations that follow it. Be sure to review the explanations for questions you got right as well as for those you got wrong. This will serve as a good review of the wide range of topics covered on the exam. After completing the exam, continue to refer to the content chapters to make sure you are familiar with everything we cover in this book.

Use this game plan to prepare for test day. Then, right before the exam, relax. You can rest easier because you're ready for the EMT-Basic. With some hard work and a little forward thinking, you're going to get a great score!

Author's Note

In the early twentieth century, emergency medical care was provided by physicians summoned to the scene of a medical emergency. In the movies from this era, when someone becomes sick or injured the call goes out to "get the doctor," who always arrives in three minutes or less with his medical bag to solve the problem.

In the middle part of the century, the local fire departments, which were always called first to emergencies anyway, began to carry oxygen resuscitators in addition to the first aid kits on the engines, and would be summoned to that increasingly common occurrence, the automobile accident, to render first aid and to transport the injured to the nearest hospital. Special trucks came into being, called rescues, and began to carry more life saving equipment, including the Jaws of Life, a hydraulic rescue tool to rescue people entrapped in damaged automobiles.

Hospitals too were changing. The main entrance as the portal to emergency medical care began to give way to the emergency room, where you would find all kinds of doctors, including dermatologists and podiatrists earning extra money moonlighting there. These part-time emergency room physicians began to give way to a new specialist, the board-certified emergency specialist, whose talent lay in quickly diagnosing and treating life-threatening illnesses and injuries.

The modern emergency medical system in the United States really began in earnest with the passage in 1966 of the National Highway Safety Act. This act was helped along by the horror stories of high-speed collisions on the new Interstate Highway System, where emergency care usually was rendered by the local funeral director in his hearse. (Talk about conflict of interest!) This act provided monies to the states to create emergency medical services throughout the country. Most often this duty was given to the local fire departments, since many of them had rescue trucks anyway. In the early days, emergency medical care consisted basically of "load and go": Pick up the injured or ill person, place him or her on a stretcher, and race to the nearest emergency room with lights and sirens all the way.

Many medical providers of this time thought that there had to be a better way and began to develop emergency medical technician courses and paramedic curricula. As with anything new, there were also the naysayers. I remember one doctor in particular who told me that firefighters could never learn to take blood pressures because it was way too complicated for them. I remembered him particularly when we upgraded our volunteer fire department rescue to advanced life support status, with 30 drugs including antiarrhythmics, analgesics, and anti-anaphylactics. So much for those who thought auscultation of blood pressures to be way too complex for us rescue types.

With the support of progressive-thinking doctors and nurses in the hospital arena, and with the desire of prehospital practitioners to be more than ambulance drivers, we have developed in this country an emergency medical care delivery system that is the envy of the rest of the world. In almost every locale a person who is sick or injured can dial 911, and within minutes, trained emergency medical technicians will be on scene to assist them and see that they receive advanced prehospital care, followed by transport to an appropriate care facility. Each day, men and women in the United States, who only fifty years ago would have succumbed to sudden illness or injury, leave hospitals alive and well, due to quick intervention by trained emergency medical technicians.

One of the noblest goals of a human being is to commit himself or herself to the alleviation of suffering. It is what drives many to enter the ranks of prehospital emergency medicine. As you prepare for your National Registry or state licensing exam with this text, we, the practitioners of this craft, prepare to welcome you as the next generation of those special caregivers who proudly wear the Star of Life patch.

Best wishes,

Richard J. Lapierre, MA
EMT-Cardiac Director
Brown University Emergency Medical Services

| SECTION ONE |

The Basics

Chapter One: **Inside the EMT-Basic Exam**

- Qualifying for the Test
- Job Description of an EMT-Basic
- The EMT Course
- The National Registry of Emergency Technicians (NREMT) Exam
- State Licensing Exams
- EMT-Basic Test Strategies: It's Not Always How Much You Know
- Test Mentality
- Kaplan's Top 10 EMT-Basic Tips
- On Test Day
- For More Information

Congratulations on your decision to become an EMT-Basic. While you haven't chosen an easy profession, it is an important and essential one, one that earns the respect of the communities you serve. While no one really wants to need your services, you will be one of the most welcome sights in any emergency. In this chapter, we'll look at the test that can get you this rewarding job.

QUALIFYING FOR THE TEST

Not everyone can become an EMT-Basic. In addition to the proper frame of mind and desire, there are also educational and physical standards that must be met. The following is one functional job description for an emergency medical technician.

Job Description of an EMT-Basic

The candidate must be at least 18 years of age at the time of the licensing examination. Generally, the knowledge and skills required show the need for a high school education or equivalent. The candidate must have the ability to communicate verbally via telephone and radio equipment; ability to lift, carry, and balance up to 125 pounds (250 with assistance); ability to interpret written, oral, and diagnostic form instructions; ability to use good judgment and remain calm in high-stress situations; ability to be unaffected by loud noises and flashing lights; ability to function efficiently throughout an entire work shift without interruption; ability to calculate weight and volume ratios and read small print, both under life threatening time constraints; ability to read English language manuals and road maps; the ability to accurately discern street signs and address numbers; ability to interview patient, family members, and bystanders; ability to document, in writing, all relevant information in prescribed format in light of legal ramifications of such; ability to converse in English with coworkers and hospital staff as to status of patient. The candidate must have good manual dexterity, with the ability to perform all tasks related to highest quality patient care. The candidate must have the ability to bend, stoop, and crawl on uneven terrain; and the ability to withstand varied environmental conditions such as extreme heat, cold, and moisture. The candidate must have the ability to work in low light and confined spaces.[1]

Quite a job description! We never said it would be easy. Check the website of your state department of health for the requirements of your state. We've provided the state EMS links in Section Four.

THE EMT COURSE

Before anyone can be licensed as an EMT-Basic, he or she must have taken a minimum 110-hour EMT-Basic course modeled on the National Standard Curriculum given by the National Highway Traffic Safety Administration (NHTSA). Most state requirements exceed the 110-hour minimum. The average EMT-Basic course now runs between 130 and 150 hours and includes all of the modules in the National Standard Curriculum. These modules are: Preparatory, which includes anatomy and physiology; Airway; Patient Assessment; Medical Emergencies; Trauma Emergencies; Pediatrics; and Ambulance Operations.

As an EMT-Basic student, you should approach your EMT course as you would any post-high school course. Skills such as note taking, promptness, and attentiveness are essential to successfully completing the course. Physical skills will also be required to complete the practical skills needed for licensing and certification.

---

[1] Rhode Island Department of Health handout, *Functional Job Description of an EMT*, 2003.

The course instructors for the most part will be practicing EMTs, who have not only gone through the same type of program you are taking, but also have had the opportunity to put into practice the knowledge and skills they have learned. Listen to them carefully, as they will be a lifelong influence on your practice. Question them and you will find them more than willing to share their expertise with you.

While participating in the EMT course, attend all classes and be prepared. Follow the directions of the instructors and you will find that you will receive all of the necessary information and skills that you need to proceed to the next level, the licensing or certification exam.

THE NATIONAL REGISTRY OF EMERGENCY MEDICAL TECHNICIANS (NREMT) EXAM

The National Registry Exam is a standardized test designed to measure the competence of the prospective EMT-Basic. The exam is written and designed by a committee made up of EMS providers and other health and educational personnel; test scores are constantly monitored to assure accuracy and fairness.

What's on the Test

The EMT-Basic test consists of 150 multiple-choice questions, many of which are scenario-based. This book will provide the EMT-Basic candidate with similar types of questions and scenarios.

There are six broad subject areas to the test with the following average number of questions:

- Patient Assessment (24–30)
- Airway (24–30)
- Circulation (22–28)
- Musculoskeletal, Behavioral, Neurological, and Environmental (21–27)
- Pediatrics and Obstetrics/Gynecology (19–25)
- EMS Systems, Ethics, Legal Issues, Communications, Documentation, Safety, Triage, and Transportation (21–27)

We'll cover all these topics in the following chapters. You'll find hundreds of questions in these subject areas throughout this book and in the Practice Test. Look for the bullet points at the beginning of each chapter for the particular subjects you want to review. We've also provided a review of the anatomy and physiology tested on the exam, so you'll be prepared.

How Long Is the Test?

The test is two and one-half hours long with no breaks.

How to Apply

You can apply for the NREMT exam online or download an application at *www.nremt.org*. You can find a testing site in your state on the same website.

Scoring

An overall score of 70 percent is passing. (That means you need to answer at least 105 questions right.) When the candidate receives his or her results, the score is broken down by the elements of the test (see above). The state office also receives students' overall scores and may share them with the instructor of that particular group of students to identify those areas that are strongest and weakest.

The NREMT points out that the goal of the National Registry exam is not to rank students but to test for competence. Their website states "the only score that counts on an NREMT examination is one that demonstrates the potential EMT has met the criteria of entry-level competence. It is this score that should allow you to start a career in EMS, to continue to learn throughout your lifetime, and to serve your department, your fellow EMTs, and the public in a competent manner." For more information, see "About NREMT Exams" at *www.nremt.org*.

Getting Your Score

Your results will be available in 10–15 days on the NREMT website and you will receive your formal notification by mail in four to six weeks. If you passed you will be a licensed Emergency Medical Technician Basic and able to perform the procedures for which you have been trained in your state.

STATE LICENSING EXAMS

Not all states utilize the NREMT exam. At the time of publication, 35 states are members of the National Registry and utilize the National Registry exam for licensure as an EMT-Basic. The remainder utilize their own exams and may require both a written and a practical examination.

The advantage of NREMT certification is that it facilitates the movement of one's license from one state to another. For example, in order to be licensed in Rhode Island, a NREMT-certified EMT-Basic from Tennessee has only to successfully complete several update courses and he or she will receive a RI EMT-Basic license after completing the normal license application process. An EMT-Basic coming from a non-NREMT-Basic state must submit documentation showing that the EMT-Basic course he or she has taken meets the minimum requirements of the NREMT, then complete any required updates, and then achieve a passing grade on the NREMT written exam.

EMT-BASIC TEST STRATEGIES: IT'S NOT ALWAYS HOW MUCH YOU KNOW

Since this test is such an important milestone in an EMT's career, good test-taking skills are crucial. To succeed, you've got to get enough right answers—as many as possible, but at least 105—in the time you're allotted. Knowing the material is not enough. You have to perfect your mindset and time-management skills so that you get a chance to use your knowledge on as many questions as possible.

It's one thing to answer an EMT-Basic test item correctly; it's quite another to answer 150 of them in 150 minutes and get more than 70 percent right. And the same goes for those long scenario questions—it's a whole new ball game once you move from doing an individual scenario at your leisure to handling dozens under timed conditions.

So when you're comfortable with the content of the test, your next challenge will be to take it to the next level—test expertise—which will enable you to manage the all-important time element of the test.

The Five Basic Principles of Test Expertise

On some tests, if a question seems particularly difficult you spend significantly more time on it, since you'll probably be given more points for correctly answering a hard question. Not so on the EMT-Basic. Remember, every question, no matter how hard, is worth a single point. There's no partial credit or A for effort on the tough ones. And since there are so many questions to do in so little time, it would be against your interests to spend 10 minutes getting a point for a hard question and then not have time to get quick points from three easy ones later in the test.

Given this combination—limited time, all questions equal in weight—you've got to develop a way of handling the test to make sure you get as many points as you can as quickly and easily as you can. Here are the principles that will help you do that:

1. Feel Free to Skip Around

One of the most valuable strategies to help you finish the questions in time is to learn to recognize and deal first with the questions and scenarios that are easiest and most familiar to you. That means temporarily skipping those that promise to be difficult and time-consuming, if you feel comfortable doing so. You can always come back to these at the end, and if you run out of time, you're much better off not getting to questions you may have had difficulty with, rather than missing material you can ace, since you may not have gotten those questions right anyway. Of course, since there's no guessing penalty, always fill in an answer to every question on the test, whether you get to it or not. Remember, too, to work on those scenarios that have the most related questions, so you maximize your points.

This strategy is difficult for most test takers; we're conditioned to do things in order. But give it a try when you practice. Remember, if you do the test in the exact order given, you're letting the test makers control you. But you control how you take this test. On the other hand, if skipping around goes against your grain and makes you nervous—don't do it. Just be mindful of the clock and don't get bogged down with the tough questions.

2. Learn to Recognize and Seek Out Questions You Can Do

Another thing to remember about managing the test is that EMT-Basic questions and scenarios, unlike items on the SAT and other standardized tests, are not presented in order of difficulty. There's no rule that says you have to work through the test in any particular order; in fact, the test makers scatter the easy and difficult questions throughout the test, in effect rewarding those who actually get to the end. Don't lose sight of what you're being tested for along with your knowledge and thinking skills: efficiency and cleverness. If trauma assessment questions are your thing, head straight for them when you first open the test.

As we've suggested before, don't waste time on questions you can't do. We know that skipping a possibly tough question is easier said than done; we all have the natural instinct to plow through test questions in their given order. But it just doesn't pay off on the EMT-Basic.

3. Use A Process of Answer Elimination

Using a process of elimination is another way to answer questions both quickly and effectively. There are two ways to get all the answers right on the EMT-Basic. You either know all the right answers, or you know all the wrong answers. Since there are three times as many wrong answers, you should be able to eliminate some if not all of them. By doing so you either get to the correct response or increase your chances of guessing the correct response. You start out with a 25 percent chance of picking the right answer, and with each eliminated answer your odds go up. Eliminate one, and you'll have a 33 1/3 percent chance of picking the right one, eliminate two, and you'll have a 50 percent chance, and, of course, eliminate three, and you'll have a 100 percent chance. Increase your efficiency by actually crossing out the wrong choices. Remember to look for wrong-answer traps when you're eliminating. Some answers are designed to seduce you by distorting the correct answer.

4. Remain Calm

It's imperative that you remain calm and composed while working through the test. You can't allow yourself to become so rattled by one hard scenario that it throws off your performance on the rest of the test. Expect to find a few killer questions, but remember, you won't be the only one to have trouble with them. Having trouble with a difficult question isn't going to ruin your score—but getting upset about it and letting it throw you off track will. When you understand that part of the test maker's goal is to reward those who keep their composure, you'll recognize the importance of not panicking when you run into challenging material.

5. Keep Track of Time

Of course, the last thing you want to happen is to have time called before you've gotten to half the questions. Therefore, it's essential that you pace yourself, keeping in mind the general guidelines for how long to spend on any individual question (a bit less than one minute). Have a sense of how long you have to do each question, so you know when you're exceeding the limit and should start to move faster. Don't spend a wildly disproportionate amount of time on any one question or group of questions. Also, give yourself a minute or so at the end of the test to fill in answers for any questions you haven't gotten to.

Answer Grid Expertise

An important part of EMT-Basic test expertise is knowing how to handle the answer grid. After all, you not only have to get right answers; you also have to transfer those right answers onto the answer grid in an efficient and accurate way. It sounds simple, but it's extremely important: Don't make mistakes filling out your answer grid! When time is short, it's easy to get confused going back and forth between your test book and your grid. If you know the answer but mis-grid, you won't get the point. Here are a few methods of avoiding mistakes on the answer grid.

Always Circle the Questions You Skip

Put a big circle in your test book around the number of any question you skip (you may even want to circle the whole question itself). When you go back, such questions will then be easy to locate. Also, if you accidentally skip an oval on the grid, you can easily check your grid against your book to see where you went wrong.

Always Circle the Answers You Choose

Circle the correct answers in your test booklet, but don't transfer the answer to the grid right away. Circling your answers in the test book will also make it easier to check your grid against your book.

Grid Five or More Answers at Once

As we said, don't transfer your answers to the grid after every question. Transfer your answers after every five questions, or find the method that works best for you. That way, you won't keep breaking your concentration to mark the grid. You'll save time and improve accuracy. Just make sure you're not left at the end of the section with ungridded answers!

Save Time at the End for a Final Grid Check

Make sure you have enough time at the end to make a quick check of your grid, to make sure you've got an oval filled in for each question in the section. Remember, a blank grid has no chance of earning a point, but a guess does. Yes, it's purely bookkeeping, but you won't get the points if you put your answers in the wrong place, or if you waste time searching for the right place to put your answers. Take the time now to develop some good answer grid habits.

TEST MENTALITY

In the previous section, we first glanced at the content that makes up the EMT-Basic. Then we discussed the test expertise involved in moving from individual items to working through a full-length test. Now we're ready to turn our attention to the often overlooked attitudinal aspects of the test, to put the finishing touches on your comprehensive EMT-Basic approach.

The Four Basic Principles of Good Test Mentality

Knowing the test content arms you with the weapons you need to do well on the EMT-Basic. But you must wield those weapons with the right frame of mind and in the right spirit. This involves taking a certain stance toward the entire test. Here's what's involved:

1. Test Awareness

To do your best on the EMT-Basic, you must always keep in mind that the test is like no other test you've taken before. If you took a test in high school or college and got a number of the questions wrong, you wouldn't receive a perfect grade. But on the EMT-Basic, you can get a number of questions wrong and still get a "perfect" passing score. The test is geared so that only the very best test takers are able to answer every question. But even these people rarely get every question right. What does this mean for you? For starters, don't let what you consider to be a subpar performance on one or two questions, or even a run of them, ruin your performance on the entire test. If you allow that subpar performance to rattle you, it can have a cumulative negative effect, setting in motion a downward spiral. It's that kind of thing that could potentially do serious damage to your score. Losing a few extra points won't do you in, but losing your cool will.

Remember, if you feel you've done poorly on a scenario, even one with more than one related question, don't sweat it. Remain calm and collected and simply do your best.

2. Stamina

You must work on your test-taking stamina. Overall, the EMT-Basic is a fairly challenging, long exam, and some test takers simply run out of gas toward the end. To avoid this, you must prepare by taking a full-length practice test in the weeks before the test, so that on test day, 150 questions will seem like a breeze. (Well, maybe not a breeze, but at least not a hurricane.)

Take the full-length practice test included in this book. You'll be able to review answer explanations and assess your performance. For additional practice material, contact the National Registry of Emergency Medical Technicians at *www.nremt.org* to receive the EMT-Basic question samples it publishes.

3. Confidence

Confidence feeds on itself, and unfortunately, so does the opposite of confidence—self-doubt. Confidence in your ability leads to quick, sure answers and a sense of well-being that translates into more points. If you lack confidence, you end up reading the sentences and answer choices two, three, or four times, until you confuse yourself and get off track. This leads to timing difficulties, which only perpetuate the downward spiral, causing anxiety and a tendency to rush. If you subscribe to the EMT-Basic test taking mindset we've described, however, you'll gear all of your practice toward the major goal of taking control of the test. When you've achieved that goal—armed with the principles, techniques, strategies, and approaches set forth in this book—you'll be ready to face the EMT-Basic with supreme confidence. And that's the one sure way to score your best on test day.

4. The Right Attitude

Those who approach the EMT-Basic as an obstacle, who rail against the necessity of taking it, who make light of its importance, who spend more time making fun of the people studying than studying for the test, usually don't fare as well as those who see the EMT-Basic as an opportunity to show off the knowledge and reading and reasoning skills that the EMS is looking for. Don't waste time making value judgments about the EMT-Basic. It's not going to go away. Deal with it. Those who look forward to doing battle with the EMT-Basic—or, at least, who enjoy the opportunity to distinguish themselves from the rest of the applicant pack—tend to score better than do those who resent or dread it.

It may sound a little dubious, but take our word for it: Attitude adjustment is a proven test-taking technique. Here are a few steps you can take to make sure you develop the right EMT-Basic attitude:

- Look at the EMT-Basic as a challenge, but try not to obsess over it; you certainly don't want to psych yourself out of the game.

- Remember that, yes, the EMT-Basic is obviously important, but, contrary to what some EMT-Basic candidates think, this one test will not single-handedly determine the outcome of your life.

- Try to have fun with the test. Learning how to match your wits against the test makers can be a very satisfying experience, and the reading and thinking skills you'll acquire will benefit you in the EMS.

- Remember that you're more prepared than most people. You've trained with Kaplan. You have the tools you need, plus the know-how to use those tools.

KAPLAN'S TOP 10 EMT-BASIC TIPS

1. Relax!

2. Feel free to skip around within the test. You're in charge. Work your best areas first to maximize your opportunity for EMT-Basic points. Choose the order in which to complete questions.

3. Be alert to the fact that the answers to some questions may be found in the others on the test.

4. For scenario-based questions, choose an answer based on the information given. Be careful not to be "too smart for your own good." Your answer choices must be consistent with the information in the passage.

5. Avoid wrong-answer traps. Try to anticipate answers before you read the answer choices. This helps boost your confidence and protects you from persuasive or tricky incorrect choices. Most wrong answer choices are logical twists on the correct choice.

6. Think, think, think! The test requires that you apply your knowledge in answering the questions.

7. Don't look back. Don't spend time worrying about questions you had to guess on. Keep moving forward. Don't let your spirit start to flag, or your attitude will slow you down. You can recheck answers if you have time left.

8. Be careful transferring answers to your grid, especially if you do skip around among the test questions.

9. Don't leave any blanks on your answer grid. There are no points taken off for wrong answers, so if you're not sure of an answer, guess. And guess quickly, so you'll have more time to work through other questions.

10. Remember, confidence feeds on itself. You can do it—and we're here to help.

ON TEST DAY

It should go without saying that on the day of the test you should prepare by being totally rested, refreshed, and focused on the task at hand. Power-cramming for the exam at the last minute by going over your notes will not achieve the desired result if you haven't been studying them all along. Pulling an all-nighter just before the exam will probably also be counterproductive, plus you always run the risk of falling asleep during the exam. Here are some basic pointers:

- Arrive at the test site at least 15 minutes before the announced start time. Before entering the examination room, visit the restroom, look at yourself in the mirror, and tell yourself out loud that you are going to be a great EMT. Never minimize what a positive mental attitude will do.

- Do not bring your notes with you, as at this point they will be more of a distraction than anything else. And they are not allowed in the test!

- You should have with you a bottle of water, a watch, three No. 2 pencils, and whatever power snack you like.

- After a detailed explanation of the national exam process and how to fill out the answer sheet, you will be given the exam booklet. Do not open it until advised by the proctor. Note how much time you have and place your watch on the desk in front of you.

- Once the book is open, read through a few questions quickly to put yourself into an emergency medical technician frame of mind. Go back to question one, take a deep breath, and begin. Read the entire question and read all of the answers. If it is a scenario, try to picture it in your mind.

- Discard the obviously false answers and choose the one that best answers the question. If you are reasonably certain of the correct answer, then mark your answer sheet and move on to the next question. If you cannot choose an obviously correct answer, skip the question and move on. After you have answered all of the questions that you are reasonably certain of, you can then return to the other questions and analyze them in greater detail.

- Many times you will find the answers to questions in subsequent questions. If there was a question you couldn't find an answer to, you may find it later and then you can go back and answer it.

- If you start to feel distracted, overwhelmed, or tired, stop. Close the book, close your eyes, and try to clear your mind. Eat some of your snack and drink some water. Take two or three deep breaths and continue. If this doesn't clear your mind sufficiently, the proctor will have given directions as to using the restroom. Usually no more than one person at a time is permitted to leave. If you can do so, go to the restroom and splash water on your face again. All of this will help you refocus to the task at hand.

- Keep an eye on the time as you want to answer all of the questions.

- If you cannot answer a question with certainty, analyze it and give it your best guess. Once again, there is no penalty for guessing. *Never* leave an answer blank because you're afraid of making a mistake.

- When you are finished with the exam, go over the answer sheet and be sure that all of the questions have been answered.

COMPUTER-BASED TESTING

Starting in January 2007, the National Registry of Emergency Medical Technicians (NREMT) is transitioning from a paper-and-pencil exam to a computer-based exam. The content and format of the state-approved practical exam will not change, and candidates will still be required to pass the practical exam before taking the EMT-Basic exam.

Please note that the subject matter will remain the same as what was covered on the paper-and-pencil exam. Only the format of the EMT-Basic is changing. Comprehensive coverage and review for each subject is provided in this book.

The fee for the EMT-Basic exam will be $70, and will cover both the NREMT registration fee and testing center cost. This will be true regardless of the testing location. In most cases, exam results will be available the next business day. The results will be transmitted electronically to the NREMT as encrypted, secure data. Then the data will be posted to their website (*www.nremt.org*) and also sent to the proper state licensing agency. Registering and scheduling will also be much easier. The exam will be administered at hundreds of testing centers across the country, and in some cases, in the evening and on weekends as well. Candidates will register and pay online, and after training and state verification, candidates will schedule their exam. Those who need to retake the exam will find a significantly shorter turnaround.

How It Works

Instead of a predetermined mix of basic, medium, and hard questions, the computer will select questions for you based on how well you are doing. This is known as a computer-adaptive test (CAT). You will only see one question at a time. If you keep getting questions right, the exam will get harder. If you make some mistakes, the exam starts giving you easier problems; but if you answer them correctly, it will go back to the hard ones. Because of this format, the CAT is structurally different from a paper-and-pencil exam. You cannot return to a question once you've answered it, or skip around within a section, because that would throw off the sequence. Once you answer a question, it's part of your score, for better or worse.

Kaplan's Strategies

Using certain CAT-specific strategies can have a direct, positive impact on your score:

- Use the computer tutorial to your advantage. Spend as much time as you need to make yourself comfortable with the computer before you begin. If you click on *Help* once the exam is under way, it will count against your allotted time for that section.

- The CAT does not begin with really easy questions that gradually get harder. Because the order of difficulty will not be predictable, always be on the lookout for traps.

- A key strategy for doing well on the CAT is to perform well early on so that you quickly get to the point where you're being given the hard questions. Getting a hard question right will help your score a lot, but getting a hard question wrong will hurt your score only slightly. Thus, it pays to spend more time on those early questions, double-checking each answer before you confirm it.

- Try to avoid getting several questions in a row wrong. If the previous question you answered was a blind guess, spend a little extra time on the next question.

- The CAT does not allow you to go back to questions you've already answered to double-check your work, so be as certain as possible that you have answered a question correctly before moving on.

- The CAT does not allow you to skip questions. So if you are given a question you cannot answer, you'll have to guess. Eliminate any wrong answer choices that you can spot and guess intelligently and strategically among those remaining.

- Sometimes it's necessary to give up on a tough, time-consuming question. It's difficult to do, but let it go and move on to the next question. That's how you score points, not by agonizing over one question.

- Don't get rattled if you keep seeing really, really difficult questions. It just means you're doing very well on that section. Keep it up!

FOR MORE INFORMATION

The material on the computer-based testing is up-to-date at the time of publication. However, the NREMT may have more information on the CAT or may institute changes after this book is published. If there are any important late-breaking developments, we will post that information online at *kaptest.com/publishing*.

You can also visit the National Registry of Emergency Medical Technicians' website at *www.nremt.org*, or contact them at:

National Registry of Emergency Medical Technicians
Rocco V. Morando Building
6610 Busch Boulevard
P.O. Box 29233
Columbus, Ohio 43229
Phone: (614) 888-8920

For state licensing exams, contact your state department of health. See the list of websites in the EMT-Basic Resources section at the back of this book.

EMT-Basic Review

Chapter Two: **Well-Being of the EMT/ Legal and Ethical Issues**

- Physical Risks

- Mental and Emotional Risks

- Medical, Legal, and Ethical Issues

Prehospital emergency medicine is a tough, demanding practice. It requires not only physical strength and conditioning, but mental and emotional stability as well. As any practicing EMT will tell you, to go from sleeping or watching television to the priority response of a life-threatening situation involves the entire person of the EMT. The body's own physiological response to excitement, the dumping of adrenaline into the nervous system, affects all aspects of our behavior, physical, emotional, and mental. Therefore, it is imperative that the EMT be in peak mental, emotional, and physical condition. Before ever setting foot inside a rescue vehicle, the EMT must be medically cleared of any conditions that would not permit the practice of all elements of the EMT job description. In addition, the EMT must have taken upon himself or herself the necessary mental and emotional disciplines to perform the tasks of an EMT. Having passed the licensing exam only means that the EMT has attained the minimum knowledge necessary for licensure. It is the EMT's responsibility to be aware of all of the emotional and mental pressures that accrue during practice.

PHYSICAL RISKS

The most obvious danger to the EMT's well-being is physical danger. It is against EMS policy for EMTs to enter any scene that they believe is dangerous. The most common example used is a patient with a weapon. Such a scene must be secured by law enforcement prior to entry. While heroics are common in the movies, the reality is that entry into an unsafe scene can result in the EMT becoming a victim and complicates the response. The initial responding EMT is no longer able to function as an EMT, his or her partner must now protect the incapacitated EMT, and an additional two teams must now respond, one for the initial victim and the second for the injured EMT. Physical dangers also include environmental hazards such as electrical wires, chemical spills, and building collapses.

The EMT is also at risk for exposure to communicable diseases, such as hepatitis, AIDS, tuberculosis, and SARS. These are preventable in a number of ways, including inoculations and wearing appropriate protective devices, such as masks and gloves. The EMT must be aware of the dangers of bloodborne and airborne pathogens and be knowledgeable not only in preventing contamination, but in the proper handling of articles exposed to bodily fluids, which may be contaminated. The proper use and disposal of hypodermic needles and syringes, commonly referred to as "sharps," is paramount. One of the most common causes of prehospital exposure to pathogens among EMTs is the "dirty needle stick." Again, these are mostly preventable with proper use and disposal techniques.

MENTAL AND EMOTIONAL RISKS

In addition to the physical danger, there is also the emotional trauma that is part and parcel of the EMT career. Most EMTs will tell you the worst call they ever handled involved the death of a child. It is impossible to shrug this type of trauma off. The emotionally healthy EMT takes this trauma, processes it, with counseling if need be, and then is capable of moving on.

While every EMT has wanted to resuscitate an apneic and pulseless patient, the fact is that death and dying are situations encountered frequently in this profession. In her well-known book *On Death and Dying*, Dr. Elisabeth Kubler-Ross points out that there are five stages in dealing with death: denial and isolation, anger, bargaining, depression, and acceptance. These stages hold true not only for the family members of the deceased, but for the public-safety personnel who attend to them as well. Many people entering the ranks of prehospital emergency medicine are teenagers and young adults, whose experiences with death may be very limited. It is important for their mentors and officers to recognize the signs and symptoms of post-traumatic stress and be prepared to intervene or, in serious cases, to provide for professional psychological assistance.

The formal response to this type of trauma may be a critical incident stress debriefing (CISD). These are conducted formally by other public safety personnel within 24 to 72 hours following a critical incident and may be followed up with a recommendation for some formal type of one-on-one intervention.

Post-Traumatic Stress Disorder

The signs and symptoms of post-traumatic stress may include unexplained irritability, an inability to concentrate, difficulty sleeping and nightmares, anxiety, inability to make decisions, feelings of guilt, loss of appetite, loss of sexual desire, isolation, and loss of interest in work. Any of these that persist for longer than a few days should be considered serious.

A good defense against serious post-traumatic stress is the sharing of the emotions in confidence with one's coworkers, especially those who were part of the call and are familiar with the details, or with those who have been through something similar on other calls. Depending on the severity of the call, processing these emotions may take months, or even years.

MEDICAL, LEGAL, AND ETHICAL ISSUES

The particular state protocols under which an EMT-Basic functions will determine his or her scope of practice and standard of care. All state protocols allow EMT-Basics to perform CPR on patients who are pulseless and apneic, for example. No state allows an EMT to perform open-heart surgery on the street.

Duty to Act

The duty to act varies from state to state. However, anytime an EMT is on duty as a prehospital medical provider, there is a duty to act on any ill or injured patient he or she encounters or is dispatched to. It is not permissible under this duty to refuse to perform the appropriate interventions on a patient whom an EMT-Basic doesn't like, or who has a condition that the EMT-Basic judges is the patient's own fault.

Patient Consent

The issue of patient consent is one of the trickiest of all medical, legal, and ethical issues. It is a generally accepted legal principle that a competent individual has the right to permit or refuse any specific medical procedure. The EMT-Basic is often confronted with the victim of a motor vehicle accident who refuses to allow the application of a cervical collar, which many states require of all trauma victims with a possibility of cervical trauma. Thus the EMT-Basic now is faced with two conflicting statutes. The competent person's right of refusal will normally take precedence; however, it has been argued that a reasonable and prudent person would want the collar, and thus collars have been forced upon patients. The EMT-Basic has to be aware that such an action may well be considered assault and battery.

Expressed consent is verbal agreement to treatment by a competent patient. *Implied consent* means a patient who is unconscious, inebriated, or otherwise cannot express consent would agree to treatment as would be given to anyone in that situation.

Competency

The word *competent*, as well, causes dilemma in the emergency medical profession. It is a recognized legal fact that a person who is seriously intoxicated is not a competent person; however there is no magic standard that defines the level of inebriation that creates incompetence. The EMT-Basic is thus thrust into the position of making this important determination on the scene and setting the level of medical care.

A minor is held by most states to lack competence so that even if a nine-year-old bicycle-accident victim refuses to allow the application of a cervical collar, the EMT-Basic can overrule the wishes of the minor child, unless there is a parent on scene who objects.

Litigation and the Good Samaritan Law

It is important to know the defenses against being successfully sued in the performance of EMT-Basic duties. Paramount among these is the Good Samaritan Law. This act provides immunity against liability for someone who performs an emergency medical procedure for which he or she is trained and licensed, unless it is done in a manner that is grossly negligent.

Along with the Good Samaritan Law goes the use of medical direction. If the EMT-Basic is in doubt of whether or not to perform a particular procedure for which he or she is licensed, the first line of defense is the state protocols. After this is the use of medical control. Consulting with an emergency room physician for advice and orders for particular interventions is always the best course of action.

Confidentiality

Numerous laws and court decisions have assured the confidentiality of medical information. What is told to the EMT-Basic by a patient is confidential and is to be told only to those to whom the EMT-Basic transfers patient care. With the Health Insurance Portability and Accountability Act, commonly known as HIPAA, the demands for patient confidentiality have increased substantially, and the EMT-Basic, as a medical-care provider, is bound by these standards. Since EMT-Basic assessments are routinely carried out in a public setting rather than a closed office, this is becoming more problematic. A person with a history of sexually transmitted disease, for example, is less likely to divulge this history if his or her coworkers are milling around as an EMT-Basic does a patient assessment. It is *never* permissible to discuss a patient's history or care with anyone outside the medical community unless compelled to do so by a legal order. When using real situations, such as those which inspired many of the scenarios in this book, extreme caution must be taken in order that the patient cannot be identified.

Crime Scenes

When a medical scene is also a crime scene, care must be taken to disturb as little as possible. Documentation of patient care must also include any disturbances that were necessary for the patient's treatment and transport.

Various state laws also address when medical personnel *must* notify law enforcement officials if they become aware of certain situations. Child abuse has become the clearest case of these situations. If an EMT-Basic is aware that a child has been physically, emotionally, or sexually abused, failure to notify the proper agency will subject the EMT-Basic not only to civil, but to criminal penalties as well. Some states also provide for the notification of sudden death, gunshot wounds, spousal abuse, elder abuse, and animal bites.

PRACTICE SET

1. You are dispatched to a call for a possible over-dose. You respond priority and are advised that police response will be delayed. You arrive on scene and are directed to a bedroom at the end of a hall. Opening the door, you see a middle-aged woman sitting on a bed, surrounded by open pill bottles and an empty whiskey bottle. She is bran-dishing a large butcher knife. The correct course of action is to

   (A) Rush her and take the knife away from her.

   (B) Throw the medical bag at her head to distract her and take the knife away.

   (C) Withdraw from the room to a position of safety and request police to expedite their response.

   (D) Talk her into giving you the knife.

2. A week following the death of an infant in a call handled by you and your partner, your partner tells you that he has been having nightmares involving the death of his own children and that he is not eating or sleeping well. Your next course of action should be

   (A) Slap him and tell him to snap out of it.

   (B) Notify your immediate supervisor of your concerns.

   (C) Do nothing.

   (D) Drive him immediately to the nearest mental-health-care facility.

3. You are called to the scene of a man down with no other information. You arrive on scene, and your partner quickly assesses the patient, turns to you, and shakes his head. The patient is cyanotic with full rigor and postmortem-dependent lividity clearly present in his torso. The man's wife is anx-ious, peering into the room and asking you if he will be all right. You gently lead her into the living room and ask her to sit down. You look directly at her and quietly tell her that her husband has died and there is nothing that you can do. She initially has no reaction, then wails loudly and throws her-self into your arms, crying out, "He can't be dead; he was just talking to me!" This stage of the grief process is called

   (A) Acceptance

   (B) Bargaining

   (C) Anger

   (D) Denial

4. After discharging a patient who had been stabbed in the abdomen to the emergency department, you are removing your bloody gloves when you notice that they are torn and that the blood has gotten on your skin. Furthermore, after you wash the blood off, you notice that you have a small fresh laceration on your middle finger. What is your next course of action?

   (A) Wash your hands again and that will take care of any contamination issues.

   (B) Disinfect the wound with hydrogen peroxide and dress it with a sterile dressing.

   (C) Immediately begin taking a mixture of ant-acid and syrup of ipecac to neutralize stom-ach acids and cause vomiting of any residual contaminants.

   (D) Report a bloodborne-pathogen exposure to your immediate supervisor and follow your service's protocol for exposure.

KAPLAN

5. Which of the following is NOT a function of an EMT-Basic?

   (A) Control life-threatening situations.

   (B) Assure scene safety.

   (C) Assess an injured or ill patient.

   (D) Disarm a patient with a firearm

6. You arrive on the scene of a man down call. Upon arrival you observe a male in his mid forties, lying face up on the sidewalk. He is snoring and you smell what you believe to be an alcoholic beverage on his breath. What legal doctrine allows you to begin treatment since he does not respond to your verbal questioning?

   (A) Juxtaposition

   (B) Monroe Doctrine

   (C) Implied consent

   (D) Expressed consent

7. You are dispatched to an unknown-type medical call. You respond priority and arrive at a residence. Police have secured the scene, and you enter the apartment and see a male in his fifties lying on a couch. He is semiconscious and smells of liquor. His response to your questioning is belligerent, and he repeatedly asks you to leave him alone and tells you that he is fine. He is unable to tell you what day it is or where he currently is. His breathing is rapid and shallow and he appears to be pale and diaphoretic. You should now do which of the following?

   (A) Have the patient sign a refusal form and go back in service.

   (B) Advise the patient that he may be seriously ill and continue to encourage him to allow you to transport him to a medical facility.

   (C) Drag the patient off the couch, place him in a hammerlock, and march him out to your truck for transport.

   (D) Advise the police that due to his medical condition, the patient must be transported and may not refuse due to incompetence because of suspected alcohol intoxication, and request that they assist you in placing the subject in the truck.

ANSWER EXPLANATIONS

1. C

When faced with this situation, the other solutions appear to be more heroic, however all other answers involve the EMT-Basic placing him- or herself at risk to be injured.

2. B

Your partner is exhibiting symptoms of depression and anxiety brought on by post-traumatic stress. While nothing in this scenario indicates that the stress is critical at this time, you have a duty to act and seek proper care for him. This is accomplished by notifying your supervisor of your concerns in order that proper mental health care can be obtained. The "snap out of it" approach works well only in the movies. Doing nothing may allow the situation to resolve itself, but it also may allow your partner to slip into a clinical depression, which will be more difficult to resolve. Driving him to the mental health facility without having done a proper workup will likely be counterproductive, much as if you were to deliver every chest pain patient to a cardiac catheterization lab.

3. D

Denial is a common first reaction to difficult news: "If I don't believe it, it didn't really happen." News of tragic importance is often accompanied by a wide range of emotions as the mind attempts to deal with information it doesn't really want to hear. As such the mind will process the emotions with whatever controls it can muster to try and delay the final stage of grief, which is acceptance. Anger may also be the first stage and the EMT-Basic often may be the brunt of the attack, both verbal and physical: "They always save the patient on television, what did you do wrong?" It is important to keep in mind that this is a defense mechanism. Bargaining serves the same purpose: "If there is something I can trade for this bad news, I will."

4. D

The combination of skin exposure to someone else's blood and an open wound could mean that bloodborne pathogens have been introduced into your bloodstream. These pathogens can include HIV and hepatitis, both of which can cause serious illnesses and are potentially fatal. Answers choices (A) and (B) deal with external exposure and will not be effective if the pathogen has already been introduced into the bloodstream. Neither will choice (C), which will cause vomiting of the stomach contents but will not be effective on bloodborne pathogens. Each service is required by law to have a protocol for these exposures which includes blood testing and medical consultation for treatments to minimize the risk of developing bloodborne illnesses; however, this is only effective if implemented and the appropriate personnel are notified.

5. D

An EMT Basic is not trained or equipped to disarm a subject carrying a weapon. This is a job for law enforcement personnel.

6. C

The correct answer is implied consent. The law allows the EMT-Basic (or any medical provider) to assume that the patient, if conscious, would consent to normal medical treatments. (A) is not a legal doctrine, but merely states that one object is next to another, (B) is a legal doctrine which the United States used as justification in the early 1800's to interfere with the European colonization of Central and South America, and (D) is when the patient consciously and competently gives you permission to perform a medical procedure.

7. D

The key is that the patient does not know what day it is or where he is. These factors give you the criteria you need to overrule his rejection of a transport, since he probably lacks the competence to refuse. (A) is only correct if you are satisfied that the patient will be fine if he signs a refusal and you leave. It is always good to remember that somebody felt concerned enough to call EMS, and you should be extremely cautious in accepting a refusal from a patient who is presenting with serious symptoms. (B) is correct, but the amount of time you should spend arguing with an intoxicated patient is limited. (C) is not part of your job description and is properly done by law enforcement.

Chapter Three: **Anatomy, Physiology, SAMPLE, Vital Signs, and Moving Patients**

- Anatomical Planes
- Skeletal System
- Respiratory System
- Circulatory System
- Gastrointestinal System
- Muscular System
- Nervous System
- Skin
- Endocrine System
- SAMPLE History
- Baseline Vital Signs
- Moving and Lifting Patients

As a medical provider, the EMT-Basic must be familiar with the standard terminology of medical practice, including anatomical and physiological definitions. A good working knowledge of anatomy and physiology is not only necessary for the practice of prehospital medicine, but must also be utilized in communication with other medical professionals. In addition to knowing the proper names for parts of the human body, the EMT must also know the anatomical planes. This will enable the EMT to properly diagnose conditions and to communicate effectively.

ANATOMICAL PLANES

The first thing the EMT must know is what is called *normal anatomical position*. Normal anatomical position is the patient standing facing forward with arms at the side and palms facing forward. In this position, it is possible to divide the human body into sections called anatomical planes (see figure 2.1).

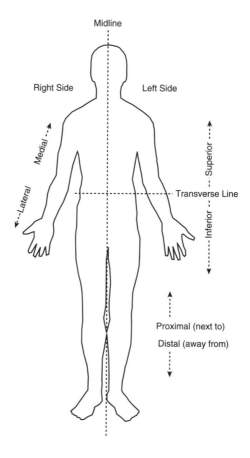

Figure 2.1 Normal anatomical position

The imaginary vertical line through the middle is referred to as the *midline*. Objects toward this midline are called *medial* and objects away from the midline are *lateral*. When working with the limbs, the terms *distal* and *proximal* are synonymous with "away from" and "next to" the trunk. *Right* and *left* refer to the patient's right and left.

So with these definitions in mind, the EMT can make the statement that the patient's right hand is proximal to the patient's right wrist and distal to the patient's right shoulder. The right wrist is also the most lateral part of the body to the patient's midline, and the shoulder is more medial. The *transverse*, or cross-sectional, line at the waist divides the body into the *superior* part ("up") and the *inferior* part ("down").

Now turn the patient to his or her side (see figure 2.2). The imaginary line from the top of the head down the middle of the torso to the feet is referred to as the *midaxillary* line. The midaxillary line divides the body into the *anterior*, or front, part and the *posterior*, or rear, part. Sometimes *ventral* is used for anterior and *dorsal* for posterior.

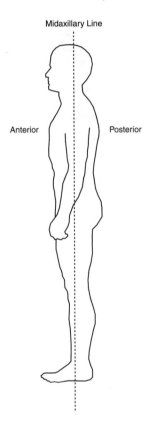

Midaxillary Line

Anterior   Posterior

Figure 2.2 Anatomical planes (side view)

So, if your patient has a stab wound to the right thigh, you could inform medical triage that your patient has a stab wound of approximately five centimeters on the medial anterior side of the right leg, proximal to the groin. This enables the nurse or physician to picture the wound on the body and plan accordingly.

Other landmarks of the body that are useful in anatomical descriptions are contained in the glossary at the back of this book.

THE SKELETAL SYSTEM

The skeleton is a collection of bones that provides the framework of the human body. The bones also provide protection for the soft tissues and internal organs.

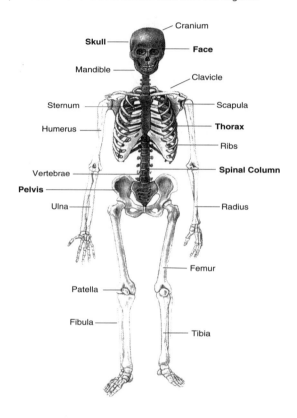

Figure 2.3 Skeleton

The skeletal system is subdivided into seven sections: the skull, the face, the spinal column, the thorax, the pelvis, the upper extremities, and the lower extremities. We will go through the bones of the system; not all are marked on the diagram.

The *skull* is basically a cap of bone that serves to protect the brain.

The bones of the *face* include the *orbit* (eye socket), the *nasal bone*, the *maxilla and mandible* (jaw), and the *zygomatic bones* (cheeks).

The *spinal column*, or backbone, is composed of a series of bones called *vertebrae*. Almost every National Registry test will have a question asking how many vertebrae compose a particular section of the spinal column. The *cervical*, or neck, section has 7; the *thoracic*, or chest, section has 12; the *lumbar*, or lower, back section has 5; the *sacral*, or pelvic, section has 5; and the *coccyx*, or tailbone, has 4. In giving locations to medical control or triage on the back of a patient, it is common to count the vertebrae to an injury and thus be able to advise medical control that an injury or pain is located at approximately T-6, for example. This location would be determined by counting the seven cervical vertebrae and then six of the thoracic vertebrae.

The *thorax* is comprised of 12 pairs of ribs, 10 of which are connected to the *sternum* or breastbone. The bottom two ribs are called "floating ribs," since they are connected in the back to the vertebrae but end before connecting—anterior. (Remember the anatomical planes; this means front). The ribs are used to locate particular locations on the chest. This is especially critical in determining the location of cardiac electrodes for cardiac monitoring. The space between the uppermost (superior) rib and the next one inferior is called the first *intercostal space*. The space after the second rib is the second intercostal space, and so on. The sternum is divided into three parts: the *manubrium,* or superior, portion of the sternum, the *middle body,* and the *xiphoid process,* which is the inferior tip of the sternum.

The *pelvis* is composed of the *iliac crests,* which are the wing sections of the pelvis; the *pubis,* which is the anterior portion of the pelvic bone; and the *ischium,* which is the inferior portion of the pelvis. The pelvis is the inferior portion of the abdominal cavity and protects the internal reproductive organs, intestines, bladder, and rectum.

The *upper extremities* comprise the *clavicle* (collarbone), the *scapula* (shoulder blade), the *humerus* (superior bone of the arm), the *radius* (lateral bone of the forearm), the *ulna* (medial bone of the forearm), the *carpals* (wrist bones), the *metacarpals* (bones of the hand), and the *phalanges* (finger bones).

The *lower extremities* consist of the *greater trochanter* (ball) and *acetabulum* (socket), which together make up the *hip joint,* the *femur* (thighbone), the *patella* (kneecap), the *tibia* (medial bone of the lower leg), the *fibula* (lateral bone of the lower leg), the *medial* and *lateral malleolus* (ankle bones), the *tarsals* and *metatarsals* (foot), *calcaneus* (heel) and *phalanges* (toes).

Where two or more bones connect is called a *joint*. There are two basic types of joints: ball and socket (hip and shoulder) and hinge (elbow and knee). Bones are connected to muscles by ligaments and tendons, which provide motion.

RESPIRATORY SYSTEM

The respiratory system provides the oxygen necessary for the body to metabolize fuel into the energies that are necessary for life. Oxygen enters the respiratory system through the mouth and nose into spaces adjacent to these anatomical devices. The space behind the nose is called the *nasopharynx*, and the space behind the mouth is called the *oropharynx* (see figure 2.4).

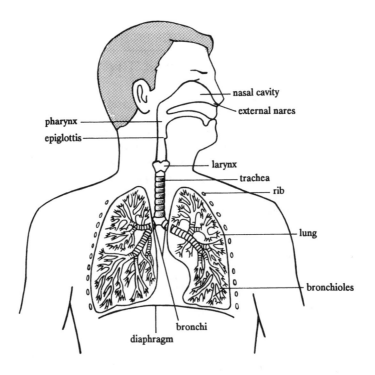

Figure 2.4: Respiratory system

At the inferior portion of the pharynx is the *epiglottis*, a leaflike valve that closes over the trachea during swallowing to prevent food and liquid from entering it. The *trachea* (windpipe) is the tube that connects the pharynx to the *bronchi*, which are the two tubes that lead into the lungs. Also considered part of the respiratory system is the *larynx* (voice box), which enables one to generate sound by passing expiratory air through the vocal cords.

The lungs expand and contract with the action of the *diaphragm* and *intercostal muscles*. As the lungs expand, negative pressure is created inside the thoracic cavity, and outside air flows into the lungs. This oxygen-rich air gives up oxygen in the *alveoli* of the lungs through the permeable walls of the capillaries and into the red blood cells. At the same time, carbon dioxide, a waste by-product of the metabolic process, also passes through these capillary walls and into the alveoli. As the lungs contract, positive pressure forces the carbon dioxide-laden air back into the atmosphere.

Respiratory Emergencies

Respiratory emergencies are a big part of the basic EMT's life, so a proper knowledge of respiratory physiology is important for diagnosis of treatable problems. Respiratory rate is often the first indicator of trouble in the respiratory system. The "normal" rate for adequate ventilation in an adult is 12–20 times per minute, for a child 15–30 times per minute, and for an infant 25–50 times per minute.

The basic EMT must also be able to distinguish between regular and irregular rates of breathing. A regular rate of breathing is where the number of breaths (plus or minus one) is the same over a period of two minutes in each 15-second cycle. Any other rate is irregular.

Breath sounds should be heard upon auscultation (listening) with a stethoscope in six separate fields: *postclavicular* (immediately below the clavicle or collarbone) on both sides (*bilateral*), *midaxillary* (just below the armpit) *bilateral*, and *subscapular* (inferior to the shoulder blade) bilateral. Absence or diminished sounds in any one or more fields is significant and must be noted.

Chest expansion should be equal bilaterally. This is determined by placing your hands over the patient's rib cage and observing your thumbs. As the patient's chest rises and falls with breathing, your thumbs should be moving evenly. As the patient breathes, the EMT-Basic must also note whether the patient is using accessory muscles of the neck and intercostal spaces in breathing. Accessory muscles come into play when the body is not receiving enough oxygen and responds by utilizing backup systems. If the patient is seated in a forward leaning position with arms forward (tripod position), this is also an important indicator of respiratory distress. This is especially significant in the pediatric population, which presents in a slightly different manner and will be more thoroughly covered in the pediatric chapter of this book. Finally, in observing and assessing respiratory distress, the EMT-Basic must note the shallowness or depth of respirations. This will usually be tied to the rate of respirations.

One important type of respiratory emergency is a *tension pneumothorax*, the complete collapse of the lung that occurs when air enters but does not leave the space around the lung (*pleural space*). It is a potentially life-threatening condition that can lead to dangerously low oxygen levels, shock, or death.

CIRCULATORY SYSTEM

The circulatory, or *cardiovascular*, system carries oxygen and nutrients to all the cells of the body. The main structure of the circulatory system is the heart, which functions as a two-stage pump and provides the life-giving action of the blood supply (see figure 2.5).

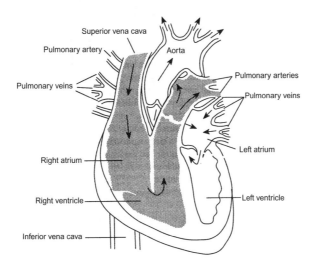

Figure 2.5 Heart

The four chambers of the heart are the *right atrium*, the *left atrium*, the *right ventricle*, and the *left ventricle*. The heart valves allow the blood to flow in the proper direction at all times. Oxygen-poor blood enters the right atrium and is then pumped to the right ventricle as the atria contract. As the ventricles contract, the blood is pumped from the right ventricle to the lungs where the carbon dioxide is exchanged for oxygen in the alveoli. As the ventricles contract and expand, the now oxygen-enriched blood is pushed back into the left atrium and then into the left ventricle and finally, with a ventricle kick, is forced into the *aorta* and into the vessels of the blood supply system.

The pump action of the heart is accomplished electrically by signals sent from the brain to the heart by the nervous system. These signals enter the superior right hand side of the heart at an electrical junction called the *sinoatrial* node (also known as the pacemaker of the heart), and pass through the atria, causing them to contract. The signal then is passed to the *atrioventricle* node and then into the right and left bundle branches of His and into the Purkinje fibers, causing the ventricles to contract and pump the blood into the lungs and into the body. This pumping action of the ventricles generates the pulse, which can be felt where arteries lie close to the surface of the skin, such as the lateral radial pulse and medial femoral pulse.

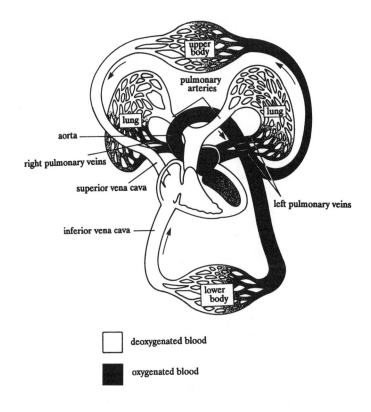

Figure 2.6 Circulatory system

The *arteries* are defined as vessels carrying blood away from the heart. The major arteries are the *coronary arteries*, which connect to the heart itself; the *aorta*, the main artery coming out of the heart, which then bends 180 degrees into the trunk and divides at the navel into the two *iliac arteries*; the *pulmonary artery*, which carries blood from the right ventricle to the lungs; the *carotid arteries*, which supply blood to the brain; the *femoral arteries*, which supply blood to the lower extremities; the *brachial arteries*, which supply the upper arms and are used to listen for blood pressure, the pressure being generated by the pumping action of the heart; and the *radial arteries*, which provide the lower arms and hands with blood. The *arterioles* are the smallest branches of the arteries and lead into the capillaries.

The *capillaries* are extremely small vessels that connect arterioles to venules. Found throughout the body, they allow oxygen to pass into the adjacent cells and permit carbon dioxide, the waste by-product of the metabolic process, to pass from the cells into the blood. The *venules*, the smallest branches of the venous system, lead from the capillaries to the veins.

The *veins* are defined as vessels carrying blood to the heart. The major veins are the *pulmonary vein*, which carries oxygenated blood to the heart from the lungs; the *superior vena cava*, which carries blood from the head and upper extremities back to the heart; and the *inferior vena cava*, which carries blood from the trunk and lower extremities to the heart.

Blood is composed of *red blood cells*, which carry oxygen, nutrients, and waste by-products; *white blood cells*, which are part of the body's defense mechanism against disease; *plasma*, the fluid component of the blood; and *platelets*, which enable blood to clot and thus stop leakage.

Hypoperfusion (Shock)

If the heart is failing to pump adequately, or there is insufficient blood to adequately provide oxygen to the cells, this is referred to as *hypoperfusion syndrome*, or shock. A patient in shock will present as pale, with cool, clammy skin, a weak pulse, shallow breathing, and low blood pressure. Hypoperfusion may also occur in patients with decreased respiratory capability. This is best measured by a pulse oximeter, a sensor that detects the infrared signature of the red blood cells from the fingernail and determines the percentage of oxygen being carried by the hemoglobin. We'll discuss hypoperfusion further in later chapters.

Blood Pressure

The pumping action of the heart is measured by blood pressure in millimeters of mercury. *Systolic pressure* is the amount of pressure measured by observing the column of mercury as the ventricles contract and the pulse is heard or felt. *Diastolic pressure* is the residual pressure in the arteries as the ventricles relax and the pulse sound can no longer be heard.

GASTROINTESTINAL SYSTEM

The hollow organs in the trunk and abdomen comprise the gastrointestinal system, the body's fuel-processing plant.

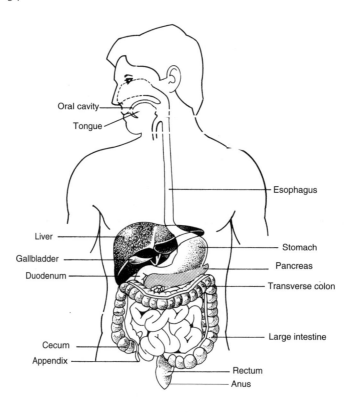

Oral cavity
Tongue
Esophagus
Liver
Stomach
Gallbladder
Pancreas
Duodenum
Transverse colon
Large intestine
Cecum
Appendix
Rectum
Anus

Figure 2.7 Gastrointestinal system

The abdomen is divided into four quadrants, with the navel as its focal point. The EMT-Basic must know which organs lie in each quadrant, since in the event of blunt-force trauma to the abdomen, the location of rigidity and tenderness will indicate which organ is damaged. The right upper quadrant contains the liver, right kidney, colon, pancreas, and gallbladder. The left upper quadrant contains the liver, spleen, left kidney, stomach, colon, and pancreas. The right lower quadrant contains the colon, small intestines, ureter, and appendix. The left lower quadrant contains the colon, small intestines, and ureter. The lower midline area contains the pancreas, small intestines, bladder, and reproductive organs.

MUSCULAR SYSTEM

The muscular system provides the body with its ability to move, gives the body its shape, and supplies protection for the internal organs of the body. There are three types of muscles.

- The first type is the *voluntary muscles*, which connect to the skeletal system and allow the body to move. The actions of these muscles are controlled by the brain and nervous system and follow the will of the individual.
- The *involuntary muscles* are under the control of the autonomic nervous system and function as necessary for the body to exist. The diaphragm, which controls breathing, is primarily involuntary, although it can temporarily be overridden by the conscious action of the person. Another example of involuntary muscles are the muscles which control the digestive process.
- The third type of muscle is *cardiac muscle*, which provides for the actions of the heart pump. While cardiac muscle is involuntary, it is unique and classified by itself.

NERVOUS SYSTEM

The nervous system is the central communications system of the body. It has two major components. The first component is the *central nervous system*, consisting of the brain, which generates all of the commands necessary for life, and the *spinal cord*, through which all signals pass from the brain to the peripheral nervous system. The second is the *peripheral nervous system*, which has two functions: *motor function*, which carries information from the brain and spinal cord to the various body systems, and *sensory function*, which relays information from the body back to the brain.

SKIN

The skin is the largest organ of the body. It serves as the outer layer of the body and holds all else in place. It serves to protect the entire body from the environment and outside organisms. Its sensory functions provide the central nervous system with most of the data necessary for the brain to function appropriately and help the autonomic nervous system to properly regulate the body's temperature, which is crucial to cellular metabolism.

The skin is composed of three main layers: the *epidermis*, or outermost layer; the *dermis*, which is a deeper layer containing sweat and sebaceous (oil-producing) glands, hair follicles, capillaries, and nerve endings; and the *subcutaneous layer* below the dermis.

ENDOCRINE SYSTEM

The endocrine system provides the body with the chemicals necessary for all bodily functions, such as insulin, adrenaline, and gender-specific hormones. The main glands of the endocrine system are the *thyroid gland*, which controls metabolism and is located in the anterior neck; the *parathyroid glands*, which produce parathyroid hormone (PTH) for the metabolism of calcium and phosphorus in the bones and are located posterior to the thyroid gland; the *adrenal glands*, which produce the adrenalin and norephinephrine used by the nervous system and muscles to control energy and response; the *gonads* (*testes* and *ovaries*), which produce the sex hormones and are located in the groin; the *islets of Langerhans*, which produce insulin to allow the body to metabolize sugar and are located on the superior pancreas; the *pituitary*, or master gland, which secretes hormones to control multiple body functions, including growth, and is located on the inferior side of the brain. (See figure 2.8.)

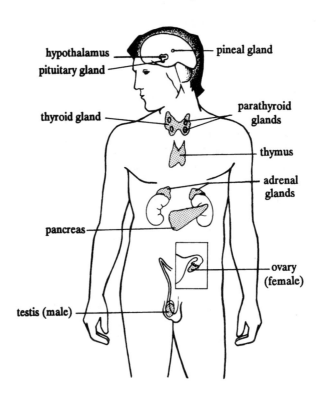

Figure 2.8 Endocrine system

SAMPLE HISTORY

It's your first time on duty, and you're wearing your new uniform shirt with that brand new EMT patch on the shirtsleeve. You've completed the truck check and now you're ready. The radio on your belt beeps, and you're about to respond to your first call. Like the rest of us, you may be experiencing fear, anticipation, and a big adrenaline rush. The dispatcher begins to speak and tells you the information that he or she has received: the address, the nature of the call, and other information that could be helpful. (Experience may teach you to take the dispatch with a grain of salt—there's the story of the EMT dispatched to a college dorm basement for a "man executed." As he repeated the call back to dispatch, the dispatcher realized her error and corrected herself to "man electrocuted." It does change the response.)

When you arrive on the scene and make sure the scene is safe, you are confronted with at least one patient. Try to avoid tunnel vision and take the time to scan the entire area, as it may affect your treatment. Step quickly to the patient, approaching from the feet if possible. The first duty is to determine if this is a trauma or medical call. If trauma is indicated or you cannot rule it out, you have to stabilize the cervical spine by taking the head in your hands. Next you have to determine consciousness. This is usually done by simply saying, "Hi, my name is Rick and I'm an EMT; what's your name?" Any response by the patient immediately tells you that he or she has an airway, is breathing, and almost certainly has a pulse. We'll assume for now that this is a medical call and that the patient is conscious and responsive (we'll deal with other assessment situations later).

The next question is usually the most helpful, and each EMT develops his or her own method of asking it, but it boils down to "Why are we here?" or "What's the matter?" Your goal is to have the patient tell you in his or her own words what the problem is so that you can deal with it as completely and correctly as possible. Once the immediate problem is stated, you want to ask six questions that will help you to get a better picture. This is called the **SAMPLE** history. **SAMPLE** stands for **S**igns and symptoms, **A**llergies, **M**edications, **P**ertinent history, **L**ast oral intake, and **E**vents leading to this episode.

Let's take the example of a female patient who tells you she has abdominal pain. Your next questions to gain information on signs and symptoms should be:

- Is it like anything you've had before?
- Can you point to exactly where it hurts?
- Is there anything that makes the pain better or worse?

Focus your questions on the multiple causes for female abdominal pain, which may include gastrointestinal problems, vascular problems, and gynecological conditions. For example, if your patient tells you that about an hour ago she developed a sharp pain in her right lower quadrant and she is holding her hand on the right lower abdomen just superior to the right leg, you may want to suspect appendicitis. Don't assume, however, and be thorough and ask the remainder of the questions.

Allergies are the **A** in **SAMPLE:**

- Do you have any allergies?

This is pretty straightforward, and people are usually willing to share this.

Next comes our **M, M**edications.

- Are you on any medications?

Now we're getting into confidential areas. Some people will give you a negative answer and then, in the privacy of the emergency room, tell the nurse the truth. This is especially true for medications for sexually transmitted diseases.

The **P** in **SAMPLE** stands for **P**ertinent history

- Are you being treated for any medical conditions?

If your female patient with abdominal pain tells you at this point that she has a history of ulcerative colitis, this may cause you to rethink your assumption that her lower right quadrant pain is caused by appendicitis. Again, certain conditions may cause patients to not tell you the truth. Be alert for signs of lying, such as the inability to maintain eye contact or a sudden change in demeanor. If you think that the patient is telling a serious lie, be sure to share your suspicions with the triage nurse at the emergency room. The goal here is not to catch someone in a lie, but to be sure that a true clinical picture emerges for the physician who will treat your patient.

The **L** in **SAMPLE** is **L**ast oral intake.

- When and what did you last eat?

If her answer is "I had two large orders of extra-superhot hot wings a few hours ago," you might want to consider that her gastric pain may be caused by indigestion.

Finally, the **E** in **SAMPLE** stands for **E**vents leading to this episode.

- What happened just prior to the pain starting?

This may give you a clue to the current condition. A person experiencing chest pain who responds to your question with "I was lifting weights" gives you a lot of information that may explain why he is experiencing this particular type of pain. While dispatches for chest pain always cause the EMT to think of cardiac-related conditions, in this case, and in the absence of any other cardiac symptoms, the problem may be a pulled muscle caused by exercising.

BASELINE VITAL SIGNS

With the **SAMPLE** history out of the way and no indications of immediate treatment needed, we can now proceed to take baseline vital signs. The baseline vital signs include: level of consciousness, pulse rate; respiratory rate and depth; blood pressure; skin condition; capillary refill; pupil reactivity, size and accommodation; and pulse oximetry.

Level of consciousness is usually determined by asking three questions and recording whether the answers are appropriate. Each EMT usually develops his or her questions over their career. Good questions to ask patients is whether they know where they are, whether they know what day it is, and if they know what happened to bring them to this situation. If the answers to the three questions are satisfactory, then it is said that the patient is *conscious*, *alert*, and *oriented times three*. If the patient is unable to state what happened, then the notation would be "conscious, alert, and oriented times two with confusion as to present event."

Pulse rate in an adult patient is usually measured by finding the pulse at the point where the radial artery crosses the wrist bone, counting the number of beats for 15 seconds, multiplying by four. If the pulse is irregular, the EMT-Basic must count the pulses for a full minute and note that it is irregular.

Respiratory rate is calculated by either placing your hand over the patient's diaphragm or asking the patient to place his or her hand there, then watching the rise and fall for 15 seconds, and then multiplying by four. As with the pulse, if the rate is irregular, take the measurement for a full minute. The EMT also should note if the breathing is shallow, deep, or labored, or if he or she can hear noises as the patient breathes, such as wheezing, snoring sounds, or barking dog sounds, all of which indicate potentially serious medical problems.

Blood pressure is usually measured by placing a blood pressure cuff (sphygmomanometer) on the upper arm and listening with a stethoscope over the inside of the elbow. The cuff is inflated to 200 mm of mercury, and then the pressure is slowly released. The point at which the pulse sound begins to be heard is the systolic blood pressure, or the pressure in the arteries as the ventricles in the heart contract and push blood into the system. As the pressure in the cuff continues to drop, the sound grows louder and then begins to diminish. When the sound cannot be heard any longer, diastolic pressure, or the pressure in the arteries while the ventricles are at rest, is taken.

In documenting *skin condition*, you want to note the skin color, temperature, and condition. The color of the skin indicates many things and is often the most useful diagnostic tool available to the EMT. Is the patient pale, cyanotic (bluish), flushed (red), or jaundiced (yellow)? This determination becomes more problematic in the nonwhite population. Is the patient's skin cool, normal temperature, or warm to the touch? Is the skin dry, or is the patient sweating (diaphoretic)? When you are dispatched to a "chest pain" call and walk into the kitchen and see an overweight male seated in a chair in pain, having difficulty breathing, and with skin that has a grayish pall, you immediately shift into high gear.

Capillary refill is a measure of how the patient is perfusing, or how well oxygen is being transferred from the red blood cells to the tissues. It is measured by depressing the nail bed and noting how many seconds elapse before the color returns. Pulse oximetry measures the same thing, but provides you and the triage team at the emergency room with an objective measurement of perfusion. If you have a patient in respiratory distress and you intervene with oxygen as allowed by your protocols, and you haven't measured the baseline perfusion, then treatment may be delayed at the emergency room while they remove the patient from supplemental oxygen to get a baseline reading on room air.

Checking a patient's pupils will often give you a good idea of his or her nervous system condition. Shine a pocket flashlight into each eye and note whether or not the pupil contracts and then dilates as you move the light out of the pupil. You also want to note whether the pupils are of equal size and whether the patient can follow the light with his or her eyes.

MOVING AND LIFTING PATIENTS

Identifying and treating patients is always seen as the main goal of prehospital emergency medicine. However, extricating patients from the circumstance that you find them in and transporting them to an appropriate medical facility is often where the real art of this type of medical practice shows through.

When lifting a patient, always do so safely. This requires exact communication with all of those involved. Before attempting to lift a patient, be sure you and your partners have a plan as to how this will be accomplished. For example, if you are moving a patient from a hospital bed to a stretcher, it is often easier to accomplish this by sliding the patient on the sheets of the bed right onto your stretcher. If there are multiple sheets beneath the patient, be sure that you all know whether you are taking all of them, or just the top one. It is critical when lifting a patient secured to a backboard or even in raising the stretcher from its lowered position to the transport position that the lifting be done in a coordinated manner. Failure to do so may tip the patient right off the stretcher and complicate his or her injuries.

When lifting a patient from a low to a high position, either on a board or on a stretcher, always use your legs to lift, not your back. This necessitates squatting to a kneeling position and keeping the weight close to your body. Your feet should be far enough apart to give you good balance in both squatting and standing positions. You should grip the stretcher, backboard, or sheets with both hands, using the entire hands and not just the fingers.

The EMT must know his or her own limitations. If the patient weighs more than can safely be handled by the crew on the scene, additional help must be summoned. Remember, all patient transfers must be done with the safety of the crew and patient as a primary consideration.

Types of Patient Transfers

There are three types of patient transfers: emergency, urgent, and nonurgent. Furthermore, each type of transfer can be subdivided into two more categories, trauma and nontrauma.

An emergency transfer occurs when speed is the primary consideration, since the patient and rescuer are in immediate danger. The most common example of this is when a motor vehicle has been involved in an accident, the driver is behind the wheel and unconscious, and the vehicle is on fire. The usual precautions for cervical spine stabilization are secondary to removing the patient from the immediate danger. This type of extrication is accomplished by whatever means removes the patient from the danger as quickly as possible. If the patient is not entrapped, grabbing the patient beneath the arms and pulling headfirst, trying to cradle the head and neck against your torso as you do so, is the best method.

An urgent extrication occurs when the situation is unstable but not critical. In the same scenario as above, but with only smoke issuing from the engine compartment and no fire visible, you may have time to take some precautions to minimize spinal injury. One EMT should attempt to stabilize by holding the head from the rear, if possible, while the second EMT applies a cervical collar. Then, with coordinated motion, the EMTs should pivot the patient so that he or she may be pulled from the vehicle by the long axis of the body onto a spine board, which can be placed right on the seat of the vehicle (if possible) to minimize patient motion. Once the patient is on the spine board, the patient can be moved away from the vehicle to a safe place as quickly as possible and receive the appropriate treatments.

In the nonurgent extrication, when there is no discernible danger, this patient would be stabilized in a Kendrick Extrication Device (see photo in chapter seven) or a similar type of stabilization device prior to being extricated.

The main piece of equipment used to effect transfers and lifting is the main ambulance stretcher, which is an adjustable-height stretcher. This stretcher comes in three configurations:

- The single-person-loading stretcher. This stretcher allows one person to place the stretcher from its uppermost position into the ambulance, as the wheeled undercarriage folds in by itself.
- The one-and-a-half-person-loading stretcher. This stretcher has a wheel assembly at the head of the stretcher, so that once it is engaged inside the truck, it enables one person to lift the stretcher and patient. The second person only has to lift the undercarriage to its resting position beneath the stretcher
- The two-person-stretcher, which requires two EMTs to stand on the side of the stretcher and lower it to the low position. Two EMTs then lift the stretcher into the truck and together roll it into place.

The other important piece of transfer equipment used by EMS is the stair chair, or folding stretcher. It is not always possible to get full-size ambulance stretcher to the patient, so the stair chair is brought to the patient and the patient is secured in a sitting position and carried to a place where he or she then can be transferred to the main stretcher.

Sometimes a patient cannot be placed in a sitting position, such as a patient who has suffered a back or neck injury. This patient must be secured to a backboard and transported on this board to the main stretcher.

PRACTICE SET

1. The patella is located in which anatomical plane?

   (A) Inferior/posterior

   (B) Inferior/anterior

   (C) Superior/posterior

   (D) Superior/anterior

2. The direction away from the midline in anatomical position is

   (A) Distal

   (B) Medial

   (C) Lateral

   (D) Proximal

3. Another name for the mandible is the

   (A) Cheekbone

   (B) Jawbone

   (C) Nose

   (D) Eye socket

4. Another name for the pelvic floor is the

   (A) Wing

   (B) Greater trochanter

   (C) Iliac crest

   (D) Ischium

5. How many vertebrae are located in the thoracic section of the spine?

   (A) 6

   (B) 12

   (C) 18

   (D) 19

6. In respiratory inspiration, air passes through the pharynx into the

   (A) Nasopharynx

   (B) Oropharynx

   (C) Trachea

   (D) Esophagus

7. You are dispatched to a residence for a female patient with difficulty breathing. You respond priority and arrive on scene to find a fifty-year-old female seated in a kitchen chair, hunched forward, pale and diaphoretic. She is breathing at a rate of 30 breaths per minute and does not have enough air to respond to your questions. A rate of 30 breaths per minute is called

   (A) Tachypnea

   (B) Apnea

   (C) Bradypnea

   (D) Crohn's disease

8. Which of the following is not a part of the respiratory system?

   (A) Aorta

   (B) Nasopharynx

   (C) Trachea

   (D) Alveoli

9. Which of the following is not a type of muscle?

   (A) Voluntary

   (B) Involuntary

   (C) Cardiac

   (D) Pulmonary

10. Which type of muscle would be responsible for the digestion of food in the gastrointestinal system?

    (A) Voluntary

    (B) Involuntary

    (C) Cardiac

    (D) Pulmonary

11. Which of the following is NOT a function of the peripheral nervous system?

    (A) Transmits information from the central nervous system to the muscles

    (B) Receives information from the senses for the central nervous system to act on

    (C) Transmits information from receptors to the brain

    (D) Processes information received from the sensory organs and orchestrates the appropriate action

12. Which is NOT a function of the skin?

    (A) Helps to regulate body temperature

    (B) Protects the body's organs from the environment

    (C) Houses the sensory nerves

    (D) Prevents the internal organs from bacteria

13. The main artery coming from the left ventricle is called the

    (A) Aorta

    (B) Nasopharynx

    (C) Trachea

    (D) Alveoli

14. Deoxygenated blood enters which heart chamber from the vena cava?

    (A) Right atrium

    (B) Left atrium

    (C) Right ventricle

    (D) Left ventricle

15. The focal electrical site that causes the ventricles to contract is called the

    (A) Sinoatrial node

    (B) Atrioventricle node

    (C) Purkinje node

    (D) Node of His

16. Hypoperfusion syndrome is best described as

    (A) Low blood supply to the tissues

    (B) High blood supply to the tissues

    (C) Low carbon dioxide output from the tissues

    (D) High carbon dioxide output from the tissues

17. Which gland is most affected by diabetes?

    (A) Adrenal

    (B) Pituitary

    (C) Islets of Langerhans

    (D) Testes

18. You are dispatched as the second rescue to a motor vehicle accident, car versus truck. You respond priority and arrive on scene. Parking the vehicle as directed by the police on scene, you see a large dump truck stopped in the travel lane and a large four-door sedan that has driven into the back of the truck. EMS personnel from the first rescue on scene have packaged the driver of the car into a Kendrick Extrication Device, extricated him from the vehicle, and placed him on a long spine board with a cervical collar and head blocks. They advise you that the patient was unrestrained at the time of the crash. The patient is conscious, but is unable to tell you what happened or what day it is. He is able to state his name and address and wants you to notify his wife. He is complaining of left side pain, left arm pain, and head pain. A glance into the interior of the car reveals that the windshield is intact; however, the steering wheel is bent. You place the patient inside your vehicle and begin a secondary trauma assessment. His vital signs are BP 100/60, pulse 90, respirations 24, SpO2 96 percent. His pupils are equal and reactive to light, and he has a laceration to his forehead with little bleeding. There are no signs of fluid in his eyes, nose, ears, or mouth. His neck is normal, with no signs of tracheal shift. You cut his shirt off and notice the imprint of the steering wheel on his chest, as well as a large bruise in the upper left abdominal quadrant. Palpation of his

chest is unremarkable. The upper left abdominal quadrant is tender and slightly rigid and the other abdominal quadrants are soft with no tenderness or rigidity. The rest of the trauma survey is unremarkable. What injury should you suspect?

(A) Ruptured appendix

(B) Tension pneumothorax

(C) Lacerated liver

(D) Ruptured spleen

19. You are dispatched to a restaurant to assist a patient with difficulty breathing. You respond priority and arrive on scene to find a female patron seated at a table hunched forward and in obvious distress. She has an airway, is breathing, and has a rapid pulse. You ask her what's happening and she states she is having trouble breathing. You ask what prescription medications she is currently taking and she tells you she only takes oral birth control pills. You ask if she has any medical problems that she is being treated for and she answers "No." You ask what she last ate and she replies that she just started eating shrimp primavera. You then ask what she was doing just prior to her having difficulty breathing and she replies, "Nothing, I was just eating." What element of the SAMPLE survey did you forget that would make a big difference in treating this patient?

(A) Allergies

(B) Level of consciousness

(C) Medical history

(D) Events leading up to this occurrence

20. The "L" in SAMPLE stands for

(A) Last Menstrual Period

(B) Last Medical Examination

(C) Last Vital Sign Readings

(D) Last Oral Intake

21. Asking a patient if there is some movement that causes a pain to increase or decrease is part of which section of the SAMPLE survey?

(A) Signs and symptoms

(B) Pertinent history

(C) Last oral intake

(D) Events leading up to this occurrence

22. You respond priority to a call for a patient in his residence who is not feeling well. You arrive on scene to find the scene secured. You see a patient sitting in his recliner appearing to be having difficulty breathing. You introduce yourself and your partner and ask him his name. He says his name is "Jim Johnson." He denies having any medical problems or symptoms. You ask him if he knows what day it is and he replies without hesitation that "It's Sunday," which is correct. You ask him where he is and he tells you that he's in the weight room at Gillette Stadium. You ask him why he thinks somebody called EMS to the scene and he tells you that he has to get ready for the kickoff. Which of the following statements best describes the patient's level of consciousness?

(A) Conscious, alert, and oriented times three

(B) Totally unconscious

(C) Conscious but not alert or oriented

(D) Conscious and alert, oriented to time, but disoriented to places and events

23. A blood pressure of 200/160 is considered

(A) Hypotensive

(B) Hypertensive

(C) Normal

(D) Critical

24. In treating a patient with "crushing chest pain," you take his radial pulse. In 15 seconds you count 22 pulses; however, you notice that the pulse is irregular. You take it again and in 60 seconds you count 120 pulses. The patient's correct pulse rate is

    (A) 80
    (B) 88
    (C) 100
    (D) 120

25. You are called to the fifth floor of an apartment house for an unknown-type medical call. There is no elevator, and you climb four sets of narrow stairs to reach the apartment. You arrive on scene, determine that the scene is safe, and enter. After conducting your primary and secondary assessments, you determine that you have an unconscious patient, possibly from hypoglycemia. There is no indication of any trauma. Which transport device would you use to transfer your patient to the truck?

    (A) Backboard
    (B) Ambulance stretcher
    (C) Crane
    (D) Stair chair

26. Precise communication with your partner(s) is crucial when affecting transfer for which of the following?

    (A) Prevention of further injury to the patient
    (B) Prevention of injury to the EMTs performing the transfer
    (C) The appearance that the patient is in capable, professional care
    (D) All of the above

ANSWER EXPLANATIONS

1.   B

This question tests not only the prospective basic EMT's knowledge of the anatomical planes, but also knowledge of correct anatomical names. Once you have determined that the patella is the kneecap, you then can place it on the front (anterior) side of the leg, which is inferior to the horizontal midline of the body.

2.   C

Distal does mean away from, but since the midline is the point in question, the correct answer is lateral. *Medial* means towards the midline and *proximal* means next to. It is helpful to remember the pairs, such as lateral/medial, superior/inferior, etc., rather than try to memorize them individually.

3.   B

While in common usage the names listed in the answers are satisfactory, the medical world requires the basic EMT to be more precise and to communicate in the manner of the profession. It is necessary for the EMT-Basic to know the correct anatomical names of the structures she or he deals with. The cheekbone is the zygomatic bone, the nose is not a bone, but consists of cartilage, and the eye socket is the orbit. A good way to learn anatomy is to purchase an anatomy coloring book. This is a preferred method of most medical students to reinforce their learning of anatomy.

4.   D

The pelvic wing and iliac crest are synonymous, and the greater trochanter is the head of the femur, which is part of the lower extremity and not part of the pelvis. The floor of the pelvis is the ischium.

5.   B

The correct answer is 12. This is a common question on the National Registry exam.

6.   C

The nasopharynx and oropharynx are parts of the pharynx located posterior to the nose and mouth respectively. Oxygenated air then enters the trachea through the vocal cords past the epiglottis. The epiglottis closes over the esophagus to prevent air from entering the gastrointestinal system.

7.   A

The correct answer is tachypnea. The prefixes *brady-* and *tachy-* refer to slow and fast, respectively. Similarly, the terms *bradycardia* and *tachycardia* refer to slow and fast heart rate. The root word *pnea* has to do with breathing or air. The word *pneumatic* refers to something air-powered. The word *apnea* refers to the absence of air, or to the condition of a patient who is not breathing. Crohn's disease does not apply here, as it is a disease of the gastrointestinal system.

8.   A

The correct answer is aorta, which is part of the heart. The EMT candidate must have a good working knowledge of general anatomy as outlined in the textbook used in the course.

9.   D

This question is hard to figure out without actually knowing the necessary anatomy and physiology, that is, that there are three types of muscle. Most people will quickly discard (A) and (B) as possible answers because of their similarity. The cardiac system refers to the heart, and the pulmonary system refers to the lungs, but in this case the key is remembering that the heart muscle is a unique type of muscle all on its own.

10.   B

The digestive process works without our having to consciously will it. We've already ruled out (D) as an answer because we know from the prior question that it's not a muscle. We know that cardiac means "heart," so we're left with involuntary and voluntary, and since involuntary is a better match for the digestive process, it's the correct answer.

11. D

These all are from the definitions of the functions of the peripheral nervous system. Note that answer (C) is the same as answer (B), slightly rephrased and with different terminology, but the same meaning. This is why it is important to read the question and all of the possible answers carefully.

12. D

(A), (B), and (C) are all functions of the skin. Bacteria are present in the organs and are used in many of the metabolic processes.

3. A

This is an example of using a prior question to reinforce knowledge, plus process of elimination. Even if the EMT candidate is not 100 percent sure of the terminology, if he or she goes back to the earlier question about the respiratory system, he or she can deduce that the last three are parts of the respiratory system, leaving the aorta the correct answer by default.

14. A

The answer is the right atrium. The anatomy of the heart is critical for the EMT to know, due to the number of emergency medical calls involving chest pain and cardiovascular problems.

15. B

Even if you get a total memory meltdown on the electrical conductivity system of the heart, you can refocus and come up with the best answer by analyzing the question. Sinoatrial contains the word *atrial*, which refers to the atrium, or upper part of the heart, so we can rule that one out. There is no such thing as the Purkinje node or Node of His; however, after the electrical command passes through the atrioventricle node, it then passes through the Bundle of His into the Purkinje fibers. The only answer that contains the word *ventricle* is atrioventricle, giving a high probability that this is the correct answer.

16. A

Again, even if we can't recall the term exactly, we can analyze the question to see which answer fits the best. First, take a look at the prefix *hypo-* which means "below" or "lower." The phrase *hypodermic needle*

refers to a delivery system that injects drugs below the skin, hence *hypodermic*. The prefix *hyper-* refers to "more" or "higher." This term is used commonly to denote a child who is overactive. Using this process, we can now eliminate answers (B) and (D). Let's look at perfusion, which sounds like it has something to do with filling up with something, or merging with something. This would make more sense for blood supply than for carbon-dioxide output, so we can state with relative certainty that the correct answer is (A).

17. C

Diabetes is a disease in which the body ceases to produce the hormone insulin, which affects the body's ability to metabolize sugar into energy and directly affects the islets of Langerhans. The adrenal gland produces epinephrine (adrenaline) and norephinephrine, which affect the nervous system; the pituitary gland secretes multiple hormones that control various glands and processes; and the testes are the gonads of the male reproductive system and produce testosterone, the male sex hormone.

18. D

The location of the bruising and tenderness indicates that there is internal bleeding in the upper left abdominal cavity. The liver is located to the right and center of the upper abdominal space, and the appendix is located in the lower right quadrant. The spleen is located on the left side of the torso at the top of the upper left quadrant. While a tension pneumothorax is a possibility given the location and type of the injury, there are currently no symptoms of that condition at this time. A tension pneumothorax may develop at any time, and given the circumstances of this particular patient it is a distinct possibility, which is why constant monitoring of patient condition and vital signs is critical.

19. A

If this patient is having an allergic reaction to seafood (which is a relatively common allergy), she still could have answered "no," since allergies may change over the years. She is presenting with the signs and symptoms of anaphylactic shock, so a history of allergies would be significant. Anaphylaxis is a true medical emergency, and many systems allow the administration of epinephrine by basic EMTs in the field. If the patient had a history of asthma, she would probably have mentioned it when you asked about medical problems she was being treated for. Medical insurance information can always wait until you have completed a full patient assessment and initiated proper treatment.

20. D

The L in SAMPLE is for Last oral intake. (A) and (B) are beneficial as follow-up questions if you have a specific concern. Regarding (C), you will initially be more concerned with current vital signs, the S in SAMPLE.

21. A

If the patient tells you that he has a shooting pain in his left shoulder, to get a better picture of the signs and symptoms you may ask him if trying to raise his arm causes it to get worse or improve. Pain is a specific symptom, and its intensity is always a good indication of what the problem may be. Also be aware that this question gives you four of the six SAMPLE survey parts. If you were unsure of the answer to question 20, for example, you could use question 21 for clues, and then go back and change your answer if need be.

22. D

"Jim Johnson" is conscious and alert, oriented to time, but disoriented to places and events. He is verbal, so he is not unconscious, and he readily answers your questions, so he is alert. He would have to have answered your questions accurately and appropriately for (A) to be correct.

23. B

Again, look at the prefixes. *Hypo-* means low or beneath, *hyper-* means high. Hypotension refers to low blood pressure. "Normal" blood pressure is considered to be 120/80, so a pressure of 200/160 would definitely be considered high. While some physicians may consider a blood pressure of 200/160 to be critical, the best answer here is (B).

24. D

Since the pulse is irregular, you must take it for a full minute. This question also illustrates the danger of not reading a question completely through. If you only read the first sentence, you would jump to a quick answer of 22 times 4, or 88, and miss the elements of the question that make the correct answer 120.

25. D

The stair chair would be used. You could use the backboard, but it would make it more difficult to navigate the narrow stairs, and since there is no indication of trauma it would not be necessary. The ambulance stretcher would probably not fit into the stairway. A crane is a nice idea, but probably impractical and would take way too long to get into place.

26. D

All of these things are true about the EMT's style of communication.

Chapter Four: **Airway**

- Opening the Airway
- Airway Adjuncts
- Respiratory Assessment
- Techniques of Artificial Ventilation
- Oxygen Delivery Systems

In order to live and breathe, every patient needs an airway, a pathway for oxygen to travel from the outside environment to the alveoli, where it can enter the bloodstream to be used in the metabolic process. As the saying goes in the profession, "A patient without a patent (open) airway will arrive at the emergency department dead and leave the emergency department dead."

OPENING THE AIRWAY

The EMT-Basic's first concern in helping the patient who has an occluded or blocked airway is to open it to enable him or her to breathe. This is a lifesaving maneuver. It is a skill that does not involve purchasing expensive equipment or taking long courses. It does involve an EMT being able to diagnose an occluded airway and then using two gloved hands to open and clear the oropharynx to enable air to enter the trachea.

Once a scene is determined safe by responding EMTs who are wearing the proper protective equipment as designated by their protocols, the EMTs approach the patient (usually from the feet if the patient is lying down) and scan the area for anything that may indicate a change in the scene status or that may have caused the emergency they are responding to. If the EMTs see a stepladder tipped on its side, for example, and an unconscious male lying on his back, it can be deduced that this is a nonurgent extrication trauma situation. The EMT-Basic can walk around the patient and call out, "Hello, how are you doing?"

If there is no response, the EMT-Basic should kneel at the patient's head and take it into his or her hands to stabilize the neck, bend down over the patient's nose and mouth to see if breathing sounds can be heard or exhalations can be felt on the EMT's cheek, and watch the patient's chest to see if there is any breathing motion. If these signs are negative, the EMT-Basic's next move *must* be to open the patient's airway.

Trauma Scenario

Since this is a trauma scenario, while holding the patient's head the EMT-Basic places his or her ring and little fingers beneath the patient's head and the thumbs along the side of his head. The EMT-Basic then places the first and middle fingers of both hands beneath the jawbone (mandible) and pushes upward. This action, called the modified jaw thrust maneuver, will not only lift the mandible, but also the tongue which is attached to the structures of the mouth, pulling the tongue away from the posterior larynx. The EMT-Basic then looks into the mouth to see if there is anything physically blocking the mouth, having his or her partner remove it and begin respirations if they do not begin spontaneously. Please note that the only two concerns here are to stabilize the neck and provide an open airway and breathing. Any other problems that may be noted can and should be addressed later.

Nontrauma Scenario

In the nontrauma scenario the actions are essentially the same, except that the airway can be opened by using the head-tilt, chin-lift method. Lifting the chin using the first and middle fingers and pushing the forehead back will move the tongue away from the posterior larynx. You can then maintain this position by placing a rolled towel or blanket beneath the patient's shoulders and have your hands free to perform additional procedures.

If the airway is blocked by solids, then the airway must be cleared by removing the object if it can be seen, or by abdominal thrusts in accordance with the foreign body airway obstruction protocol. If the airway is blocked by fluids such as vomit, then suctioning may be indicated in order to clear the airway. Suctioning is accomplished by inserting a vacuum-powered tube into the larynx. Suctioning is always done as the tube is being withdrawn and suctioning is never done for more than 15 seconds at a time as the suctioning also is removing any oxygen in the oropharynx.

AIRWAY ADJUNCTS

The EMT-Basic has at his or her disposal a number of devices to assist in maintaining a patent airway and to ensure the proper oxygenation of a patient.

Once a patient has a patent airway, it can be maintained by using oropharyngeal airway or OPA. The OPA is a device that hooks beneath the tongue, holding it away from the posterior larynx. OPAs come in various sizes, and the proper one is selected by measuring from the tip of the ear to the corner of the mouth. It is inserted backward to the normal anatomical position and twisted into the proper position or inserted in anatomical position as a tongue depressor is used to hold the tongue down and the OPA is observed going into the correct position. If a patient gags as the OPA is being inserted, it should be withdrawn immediately, and another method is used.

An alternative to the OPA is the nasopharyngeal airway, or NPA. This is a soft tube that is inserted into the nasopharynx through the nose and accomplishes an airway maneuver by holding the nasopharynx open and lifting the tongue. It can be used on a patient with a gag reflex or on a patient whose teeth are clenched because of seizure or some other medical condition. The NPA is measured for length by measuring from the tip of the patient's nose to the tip of the ear. It is lubricated with sterile water-soluble lubricant and inserted into the larger nostril with the bevel toward the septum with a back-and-forth twisting motion. Once the flange of the NPA reaches the nostril, stop inserting and evaluate your patient. The NPA is contraindicated in any patient with facial trauma or possible skull fracture as there may be an opening that would allow the NPA to enter the cranial compartment.

RESPIRATORY ASSESSMENT

In order to properly assess respiratory function, it is necessary to know respiratory physiology and the signs and symptoms of respiratory pathology. This is accomplished by observing the rising and falling of the chest as the patient breathes in and out and looking for the use of accessory muscles in the intercostal spaces and neck, checking for adequate volume during exhalation by placing your cheek over the patient's mouth, determining whether the patient has enough oxygen to speak normal sentences, and finally by auscultating the lungs. Auscultation involves the use of a stethoscope to listen to the functioning of the lungs.

Textbooks differ on the best locations to listen for breath sounds. Since there are five lung lobes or sections—three on the right and two on the left—a comprehensive assessment should include all five. This is best accomplished by locating the following six anatomical landmarks and placing a stethoscope on them. The first assessment should be done on the left chest, proximal to the clavicle at the midclavicular line. Listen for the breath sound, which should be the sound of air flowing in and out without obstruction. Then move to the same spot on the right chest. Always listen to one side and then the other (bilateral auscultation) in order to compare the sounds in opposite fields. The third spot is on the left lateral chest on the midaxillary line, with the fourth on the opposite side. Finally, the fifth spot is on the left back below the scapula, opposite the midclavicular line, and the sixth spot on the right side.

Abnormal breath sounds that would indicate some type of respiratory impairment include *rhonchi*, or snoring-type sounds; *stridor*, or a high-pitched sound on inspiration; *gurgling*, which indicates fluid in the airway; *crowing*, which is caused by a narrowing of the larynx; *wheezing* sounds, indicating narrowing of the bronchioles; and *rales*, which are a fine crackling-type sound caused by fluid in the alveoli.

Once the EMT-Basic understands how to conduct a respiratory assessment, then he or she needs to know the signs and symptoms of adequate and inadequate breathing. The four criteria which make this determination are *rate*, *rhythm*, *quality*, and *tidal volume*. The term "normal" is always subject to debate and textbooks differ on what is a normal respiratory rate, some stating 8 to 24 respirations per minute and others 12 to 20. If we average out the two, a rate higher than 22 would be considered tachypnea, and a rate lower than 9 would be considered bradypnea. The rhythm is determined by noting the times of inspiration, exhalation, and pause between. They should be equal between each cycle. Quality is determined by use of the accessory muscles. If the patient is utilizing the accessory muscles of the intercostal spaces and neck in order to breathe, or is having some type of difficulty, then it must be noted. Finally, the tidal volume, or depth of ventilation, must be sufficient for the person to speak normally, and the chest should rise and fall with each breath cycle.

TECHNIQUES OF ARTIFICIAL VENTILATION

In the event of poor or absent respirations, the EMT-Basic has to perform artificial ventilation of the patient. This is accomplished by forcing air into the lungs, utilizing a technique known as positive pressure ventilation (PPV). There are three primary methods of performing PPV available to the EMT-Basic: mouth to mask, the bag-valve mask, and the oxygen demand valve.

Pocket Mask

Dedicated EMT-Basics are never too far away from a pocket mask. Most have one on their person whenever they are on duty and have one in their private vehicle, one in their house, and one wherever they tend to spend a lot of time. In order to adequately ventilate with a pocket mask, it is imperative that the mask be tightly sealed to the patient's face. This is best accomplished by making a "C" with the thumb and first finger of both hands and holding the mask with those four fingers. The remaining six fingers are then used to pull the mask to the face by placing them on the inferior side of the mandible and gripping. The pocket mask should contain a one-way mouthpiece into which the EMT-Basic can blow into the patient's pharynx at a rate of 12 to 15 times per minute. You should be able to feel the air entering the patient's lungs and see the patient's chest rise. This method is used when there is no other EMS equipment available, to sustain a patient's oxygen-saturation level until more effective ventilation can be achieved.

Bag-Valve Mask (BVM)

The bag-valve mask (BVM) is the EMT-Basic's main tool for artificial ventilation. As with the pocket mask, a tight seal between the mask and the face is necessary for the BVM to function effectively. The BVM provides a higher concentration of oxygen than exhaled air and lessens the contact with biological hazards for both the patient and the EMT. When using the BVM, the EMT uses a one-handed "C" technique as described earlier for the pocket mask. The other hand is used to squeeze the bag and push air into the patient. The BVM also comes with an oxygen inlet port, which allows the patient to be ventilated with 100 percent oxygen. An experienced EMT can feel in the resistance of the bag the efficiency of the ventilation effort, as well as noting the patient's chest rise and the exhalation of air after inspiration.

Oxygen Demand Valve

The oxygen-powered ventilation device provides the same type of ventilation, but with less physical exertion as it is not necessary to squeeze a bag to inflate the lungs. However, the mask must be sealed on the face as with both the OPA and the BVM. Many services have discontinued the oxygen-powered device as many EMTs feel that the BVM gives better control of artificial ventilation and that with an oxygen hookup, the amount of oxygen delivered with either device is 100 percent.

With the increase in communicable diseases that can be spread by intimate contact, mouth-to-mouth resuscitation has been utilized less and less in favor of the above methods. In practice, mouth-to-mouth is now used only when the EMT is reasonably certain that there is no risk of contamination.

OXYGEN-DELIVERY SYSTEMS

Oxygen is the most widely used drug by EMS and is indicated in almost all protocols for difficulty breathing, as well as many others, such as chest pain. Consequently it is carried aboard all EMS vehicles and is used routinely by EMTs. There are usually two types of delivery systems, the onboard system and the portable system. The onboard system is usually stored in an "M" cylinder, which contains approximately 3,000 liters of oxygen. Portable systems are designed to be carried to a patient, and the oxygen is stored in a smaller "D" or "E" cylinder, each of which carry 350 and 625 liters, respectively. These cylinders are filled to a maximum pressure of 2,000 pounds per square inch and must be handled with care. If heated, a full cylinder may rupture and cause an explosion that can easily kill a bystander.

In order to be used for EMS purposes, the pressure must be reduced by a pressure regulator, which is attached to the valve of the tank. This regulator can then be adjusted to provide the proper flow to the patient in liters per minute.

Oxygen is delivered to the patient either by a mask that fits over the nose and mouth, or a nasal cannula, which fits into the nostrils. Masks come in different styles, which are indicated by the percentage of oxygen called for. A full nonrebreather mask at a flow rate of 10 to 15 liters per minute delivers almost 100 percent oxygen to the patient, while a simple face mask flowing at 6 to 10 liters per minute delivers approximately 40 to 60 percent oxygen. A nasal cannula delivers approximately 20 to 40 percent oxygen at a flow rate of two to six liters per minute.

The choice of delivery device is predicated on the degree of hypoxia (low oxygen) present in the patient. A patient who presents with cyanosis requires more oxygen than a patient who is complaining of an inability to catch his breath and has normal skin color. This is where a pulse oximeter is useful in determining just how hypoxic the patient is. A patient who complains of difficulty breathing, yet presents with normal color and a pulse oximeter reading in the high 90s, is a candidate for a nasal cannula, while the pale patient with a saturation below 90 percent would probably need a higher concentration device, such as a full nonrebreather.

PRACTICE SET

1. You are dispatched to a local nursing home for a patient with difficulty breathing. You respond priority as a Basic Life Support unit and arrive on the scene. Upon entering the patient's room, you find two nurses standing over a seventy-year-old male patient lying supine in bed. His breathing is distressed and he is using his accessory muscles to breathe. The nurse advises you that when they were checking their patients they found him in respiratory distress. They also advise you that his respiratory rate is 34 and shallow, his oxygen saturation is 78 percent, and you notice that he is pale. You are wearing universal precautions and there is no indication of any scene safety issues. Your next move would be to

   (A) Place him on 12 liters per minute oxygen via a non-rebreather mask.
   (B) Open his airway using a head-tilt, chin-lift.
   (C) Ventilate the patient with a bag-valve mask.
   (D) Request an Advanced Life Support intercept.

2. You are dispatched to a residence for a child not breathing. The scene is safe, and you are wearing gloves. Entering the living room, you see a four-year-old child lying on his back and his mother standing behind the couch screaming, "My baby, my baby." You walk up to the child and take stabilization of the head, look, listen, and feel for air exchange; none is noted. You perform a modified jaw thrust and again look, listen, and feel, and air exchange is still negative. You instruct your partner to attempt to ventilate, and she advises you that there appears to be an obstruction. You reposition the airway, and she tries again with no success. Your next instruction is to

   (A) Call 911.
   (B) Examine the airway.
   (C) Have your partner perform five abdominal thrusts.
   (D) Roll the patient over and perform five back blows.

3. In the scenario in question 2, when you examine the airway, you see a small toy truck about two inches long in the back of oropharynx. What suction device would you tell your partner to use to remove it?

   (A) 14-gauge French catheter
   (B) Rigid-tip Yankhauer catheter
   (C) Untipped suction hose
   (D) Her fingers

4. The correct landmarks for sizing a nasopharyngeal airway are

   (A) Tip of ear to tip of nose.
   (B) Tip of ear to corner of mouth.
   (C) Corner of mouth to tip of nose.
   (D) Corner of mouth to tip of ear.

5. Which of the following is a contraindication for use of a nasopharyngeal airway?

   (A) Apnea
   (B) Seizure
   (C) Facial trauma
   (D) Pulse oximetry saturation reading less than 90 percent

6. Which of the following should be used to lubricate a nasopharyngeal airway?

   (A) Petroleum jelly
   (B) Olive oil
   (C) Water-soluble lubricant
   (D) 90-weight petroleum lubricant

7. You respond to a residence for a call for difficulty breathing. In the bedroom is a forty-year-old female sitting up in bed in severe respiratory distress. She is pale, and you note that her neck muscles are protruded. She is breathing at a rate of 30. You introduce yourself and your partner and ask what her problem is. She tries to say, "Can't breathe," but is barely able to get out the two words. Her pulse oximetry is 72 percent on room air, and her husband tells you she has a history of emphysema and is taking medications for it. She is not on supplemental oxygen. She has no other pertinent history and no allergies. Auscultation of her chest, sides, and back reveal the presence of rhonchi in all fields. Which of the following is the most appropriate first treatment?

(A) Administer .3 mg epinephrine SQ.

(B) Administer 325 mg aspirin PO.

(C) Administer oxygen via nasal cannula at six liters per minute.

(D) Administer oxygen via nonrebreather mask at 15 liters per minute.

8. You are transporting the patient in question 7 to the emergency room. Her pulse oximetry has risen to 92 percent with supplemental oxygen, and her respiratory rate is now down to 20 breaths per minute. Suddenly she becomes unconscious, and you notice she has stopped breathing. You open her airway and she still does not breathe spontaneously and has no gag reflex. What devices, in the correct order, would you utilize next?

(A) Oxygen-powered ventilator, OPA, NPA, suction

(B) Suction, NPA, BVM

(C) OPA, BVM

(D) BVM, NPA, OPA

9. You respond to a residence for a call for difficulty breathing. You enter the bedroom of a sixty-year-old female, seated with her shoulders hunched forward in respiratory distress. Her pulse oximetry is 78 percent, her respiratory rate is 30, and she is pale and diaphoretic. Auscultation of the lungs reveals a crackling-type sound in the posterior bases. This type of sound is referred to as

(A) Rales

(B) Rhonchi

(C) Crowing

(D) Wheezing

10. In the scenario in question 9, which of the following is the most correct immediate intervention?

(A) Lie the patient down and perform an airway maneuver.

(B) Request an ALS intercept.

(C) Administer five abdominal thrusts to clear the airway.

(D) Administer oxygen 15 liters per minute via nonrebreather mask.

11. While attempting to ventilate a patient who has stopped breathing while en route to the hospital, you insert an OPA and place a BVM over the patient's mouth and nose and squeeze the bag. You note that there is not much resistance and that the patient's chest does not rise. Which of the following is the most likely cause of this failure?

(A) Inadequate oxygen supply

(B) Equipment failure

(C) Failure to pre-oxygenate the patient

(D) Failure to seal the mask against the patient's face

12. In the scenario in question 11, which method is NOT an approved method of inserting an OPA?

    (A) Reverse anatomical position and twist

    (B) Normal anatomical position with tongue depression

    (C) Positive abdominal thrust with anatomical placement

    (D) Reverse anatomical position and rotate into anatomical placement

13. While conducting your truck check at the beginning of your shift, you notice that the onboard oxygen system tank has no pressure left. What size tank should you replace it with?

    (A) D

    (B) E

    (C) M

    (D) X

ANSWER EXPLANATIONS

1. B

After assuring that the scene you are entering is safe and that you are wearing universal precautions, your next step in the medical scenario is *always* to assure that your patient has a patent airway. The other options are all treatments that you may wish to consider once you have established a patent airway for the patient.

2. B

The patient may have aspirated a foreign object, causing the airway blockage. If you cannot see anything obstructing the airway, then have your partner perform the five abdominal thrusts as per the protocols for foreign-body obstruction in a four-year-old. (A) is not correct because you *are* 911, although you may want additional help or an ALS intercept. (D) is not currently the protocol for this age group, in addition to the chance of compounding possible spinal cord injury.

3. D

A blockage of this type can be removed by grasping it with two fingers and removing it from the airway. (A), (B), and (C) are all suction devices designed for fluids, which will probably be ineffective in removing an object as large as this.

4. A

The correct answer is (A). (B) and (D) are the correct answers for an oropharyngeal airway, and (C) is not used for any airway device.

5. C

Facial trauma contraindicates use of the nasopharyngeal airway due to the possibility of an opening into the cranium that would allow the device to penetrate into that compartment and complicate the fracture. (A) is the absence of breathing which would indicate use of an airway adjunct to assist with ventilations. (B) often indicates the use of an NPA versus an OPA due to teeth clenching, and (D) is an indication that oxygen perfusion is needed.

6. C

(A) will break down the material of the NPA, (B) will not lubricate sufficiently and its liquidity may cause choking, and (D) is useful only in lubricating heavy machinery.

7. D

(A) is the treatment for anaphylaxis (allergic reaction), and (B) is a treatment for chest pain. The key to the remaining answers is in the pulse oximetry reading of 72 percent, which indicates severe hypoxia. Six liters per minute will help raise the patient's oxygen saturation, but not as quickly as 15 liters per minute. Remember that a nasal cannula only delivers a maximum of 40 percent oxygen, while a nonrebreather will deliver almost 100 percent.

8. C

The correct procedure in this situation is to provide artificial ventilation to the patient. Once you've manually opened the airway, use an OPA to assist in maintaining the airway and ventilate with a BVM using supplemental oxygen. There is no indication in this scenario for the use of suction, or for an NPA.

9. A

Rales are a fine crackling sound caused by fluid in the alveoli and are usually an indication of pulmonary edema, most often caused by congestive heart failure. Rhonchi are snoring-type sounds, crowing is high-pitched sounds coming from the upper airway, and wheezing is even higher-pitched sounds coming from the bronchi.

10. D

A conscious patient with pulmonary edema will be unable to breathe if you try to lie her down in a supine position, and she will resist your efforts to do so. Pulmonary edema can be treated with ALS drugs, but your patient's immediate need is oxygen perfusion, which you can accomplish with supplemental oxygen. There is no indication of any airway obstruction, so abdominal thrusts are clearly not indicated.

11. D

Lack of resistance when squeezing the bag means that the air is going somewhere else. Equipment failure, such as a leak in the bag or mask, is a possibility, but not likely.

The percentage of oxygen and pre-oxygenation, while important to the patient's condition, have nothing to do with the physical ventilation of the lungs.

12. C

The correct answer is (C), since there is no such maneuver. An OPA may be inserted by either (A) or (B). This question requires careful reading, because the question asks for which answer is not correct, and answers A and D are identical but worded differently.

13. C

D and E cylinders are for portable use, and there is no such thing as an X tank for emergency medical oxygen.

Chapter Five: **Patient Assessment, Communications, and Documentation**

- Scene Size-Up

- Initial Patient Assessment

- Focused History and Physical Exam: Medical

- Focused History and Physical Exam: Trauma

- Detailed Physical Exam

- Ongoing Assessment

- Communications

- Documentation

It is just after midnight when your radio beeps and dispatch announces, "Rescue 1, respond to 123 Main Street, unknown-type medical call, no other information available." You pull on your examination gloves and respond priority to the call. An unknown-type medical call is a truly random event, and you can encounter something as simple as a splinter in a finger or the danger of an ongoing gun battle. Dispatchers are trained to try and get as much information as they can from a caller, but the information they are given may be fragmented or incomplete, especially if the call is coming from a third party.

SCENE SIZE-UP

Here are some guidelines for assessing the scene. Remember, this information may be critical to patient care, or even a police investigation.

Assess for Hazards

As an EMT-Basic you must be able to ascertain to the best of your ability whether a scene is safe, and you always want to err on the side of caution. You see a person down and your first inclination is to run right over and render care, but even before you get out of the truck, you must scan the area and see if there are any hazards present that would endanger your safety or the safety of your crew.

These hazards may be people who present a danger, such as a person with a weapon; hazardous materials, such as toxic or dangerous chemicals; or environmental hazards, such as unstable ground, ice, or snow. If you determine a scene is unsafe, it must be made safe before entering.

Observe the Scene

Once the scene has been made safe, you should be observant of all that is around you. This observation will also assist you in determining whether this is a medical call or a trauma call, since that determination will be important in how you assess and treat your patient. Always do the following:

- When you approach a scene, you must act as a medical detective, looking for the clues which will allow you treat this situation properly. The patient is usually the best source of information, if they are conscious and alert. If this is not the case, then bystanders become your next best source. Don't ignore the people standing around if you cannot ascertain from the victim what the problem is.

- The number of patients is also a concern that has to be dealt with immediately. The number of patients and the severity of injury or illness will help determine how many additional units will be needed at this event.

- If this is a medical call, then the nature of the illness must be determined as soon as you have established that the patient has an airway, is breathing, and has a pulse (ABC). If you determine that this is a trauma call, then you must next determine what the mechanism of injury is, or how this patient became injured. Again, ABCs must be checked first (see below).

- Do not get tunnel vision when encountering a seriously injured patient. An open femur fracture will definitely get your attention, and even if you treat it correctly with a properly applied traction splint, but forget to check for an open airway, you may deliver a dead patient to the ER with a properly applied traction splint.

INITIAL PATIENT ASSESSMENT

Remember Your ABCs

As you approach a patient, ideally from the feet, you observe him or her to determine priority, age, gender, and overall appearance. Always introduce yourself as an EMT and ask the patient his or her name. If the patient is conscious and responsive, this will tell you right away that he or she has an airway, is breathing, and has circulation (ABC). If the patient is unconscious, first check the airway, open it if necessary, ventilate if apneic, and ascertain whether there is a pulse. The rule is always to treat life-threatening situations as you encounter them. If the patient has no pulse, then CPR has to be commenced immediately.

Level of Consciousness

If the patient has no immediate life-threatening conditions, the EMT-Basic must then determine what level of consciousness exists. There are four levels of consciousness that the EMT-Basic must be able to recognize: fully **a**lert (responds appropriately to a normal voice), responsive to verbal stimuli (responds if spoken to in a loud voice), responsive to painful stimuli (responds to a vigorous rub of the sternum or an ear twist), and unconscious (does not respond). This can be remembered by the acronym **AVPU**.

Bleeding and Perfusion

With ABCs taken care of and level of consciousness established, the EMT-Basic must next check for gross hemorrhage or major bleeding. If these are present, steps must be taken to control the bleeding. Specific techniques will be discussed in the trauma section.

The next step is to rapidly determine how well the patient is perfusing, or how well oxygen is being carried to the cells for metabolism. Skin color is one of the best indicators of perfusion. In patients of color, this is more problematic; the nail beds are a better indicator of perfusion. The nail beds should also be checked for capillary refill. This is done by squeezing the nail, causing it to blanch or whiten. It should return to a normal pink color within two seconds. A delay is indicative of circulatory or respiratory distress. In Caucasian patients, pink skin color indicates normal perfusion; pale or gray pallor indicates that there is a problem. Flushed color or yellowish tinge are also indicative of problems, which we will discuss in the medical emergencies section.

Temperature

As you assess, feel the patient's forehead and exposed areas for temperature. The skin should be warm and dry. If it is hot to the touch, then the patient may be running a fever or have been exposed to high temperatures. If cold, then the patient may be hypothermic from cold exposure or have circulation impairment. Is the skin dry or moist? Dampness may be due to diaphoresis, or sweating, a symptom of many problems.

The Load-and-Go Decision

The initial assessment is performed primarily to indicate whether the patient should be transported immediately, or if there is time to perform a more thorough assessment on scene and perform any applicable treatment protocols. A patient who presents as being in serious condition should be transported immediately, with any further assessments and/or interventions done en route to the emergency room. In addition, the following are considered "load and go" patients based on the primary assessment:

- Unresponsive with no gag reflex
- Responsive but unable to follow commands
- Dyspnea (difficulty breathing)
- Hypoperfusion syndrome (shock)
- Childbirth with complications
- Chest pains with pallor and dyspnea
- Uncontrolled hemorrhaging
- Severe pain

If any of these situations are encountered, the patient should be packaged appropriately and transport initiated to the nearest emergency room. Depending on the local circumstance, the basic EMT may also consider requesting an advanced life support (ALS) intercept (if available) to initiate advanced protocols with less loss of time to the patient. Note that the primary consideration is time lost. If the ALS unit takes 20 minutes to respond and you can be at the emergency room in 15 minutes, then going directly to the emergency room without stopping is the correct call.

If at this point, the decision is that this is not a priority transport, then the EMT-Basic proceeds to the appropriate focused assessment and physical examination. *Be aware that at any time the patient's condition may change, or the focused assessment may discover a condition that necessitates an immediate transport. If this is the case, transport without delay.*

FOCUSED HISTORY AND PHYSICAL EXAM: MEDICAL

Regardless of whether you have decided to prioritize transport or not, the next step is to conduct a focused history and physical exam of the patient.

Vital Signs

Vital signs are taken at this point and include blood pressure, pulse rate, respiratory rate, and pulse oximetry. These initial vital signs are recorded and will become part of the patient's medical record.

OPQRST

Next is the assessment of the patient's complaints and signs and symptoms. The acronym **OPQRST** is helpful in remembering what to ask about the condition that has brought EMS to this patient at this time. Besides an alphabet sequence, **OPQRST** stands for:

- Onset
- Provocation
- Quality
- Radiation
- Severity
- Time

For example, you respond to a patient with chest pain. Scene safety, universal precautions, and ABCs are all done, and the primary assessment gives you no indications of a need for expediting transport. Since your patient is conscious and alert, you want to ask when the pain started (**o**nset), did he do anything to aggravate it (**p**rovocation), can he describe the pain (**q**uality), does it move in any direction (**r**adiation), how bad is the pain on a scale of 1 to 10 (**s**everity), and how long has he had this pain and has he ever experienced anything similar before (**t**ime)? If in this scenario the patient answers your questions as follows: "The pain started right after

I finished exercising an hour ago. I was lifting weights, and all of a sudden I felt a sharp pain right here [points to left chest superior to his left nipple]. If I raise my left arm, it gets a lot worse, and it feels like a tearing sensation; the pain doesn't move. I would rate it about a 6 on the 1 to 10 scale, and I've never had anything like it before." His answers would point toward an injury to the pectoral muscle during his exercising, rather than to another condition, such as a heart attack.

SAMPLE

After the **OPQRST** questions, the next assessment is the **SAMPLE** history.

- What are the **S**igns and symptoms of the medical problem?
- Does the patient have any **A**llergies?
- Is the patient taking any **M**edications?
- What is the pertinent **P**ast history of this condition?
- What and when was the **L**ast oral intake?
- What were the **E**vents leading to this situation?

If the patient is unconscious or otherwise unable to respond, then bystanders and/or family members are the best resource for these assessments.

At this point the EMT-Basic should have a general clinical picture of what the condition is and is ready to conduct a thorough physical exam. It is not necessary to palpate the entire body of a patient; however, it is necessary to physically examine the area of complaint. Palpating with the fingertips is often revealing as to what the ultimate diagnosis will be. Does the area of complaint appear normal in relation to the surrounding body areas? When you feel it with your fingers, does it feel the same as the surrounding tissue or is it abnormally rigid? When you palpate, does the patient complain that your touching is tender or painful? Remember, pain increasing or decreasing is a sign of something wrong.

At the conclusion of the focused medical assessment, if the patient is unconscious, position the patient to protect the airway, and transport the patient to the hospital emergency room. Remember that assessment is constant and be alert during the transport for changes in the patient's status and be prepared to respond accordingly.

FOCUSED HISTORY AND PHYSICAL EXAM: TRAUMA

The initial assessment will make the determination whether the patient is medical or trauma. The general rule is that unless you can definitively rule out trauma, then you are dealing with trauma.

The key in trauma assessment is to be able to identify "load and go" situations and respond accordingly. Once you have taken head stabilization and checked for the patient's ABCs and ruled out gross hemorrhage, you first must reevaluate the mechanism of injury to determine if it is significant for major trauma. Causes of the injury such as ejection from a motor vehicle, death in the same motor vehicle, falls over 20 feet, high-speed collisions, pedestrian struck by a motor vehicle, motorcycle accidents, or penetrating injuries would create an expedited transport scenario. This list is not comprehensive, nor is it meant to be, but should be used as a guide to making the "load and go" decision. In the event that the patient is under the age of 12, then falls greater than 10 feet, bicycle collisions, and medium-speed crashes would be added to the list.

The nature of trauma injuries, many of which are easily overlooked in the initial assessment, actually requires two separate assessments in addition to the initial one. The first is the rapid assessment and consists of continued spinal stabilization, airway-breathing-circulation ABCs, possible Advanced Life Support intervention, reevaluation of the rapid transport decision, and reassessment of mental status. Also note that the patient must be fully exposed to conduct this assessment. This can cause some concern, especially when the patient is the opposite gender from the EMT, but the desire to protect the patient's modesty is not a sufficient reason to perform an inadequate assessment. Protection of modesty must be a concern, however, and should be accomplished as necessary without jeopardizing the patient's assessment.

DCAP-BTLS

As each area of the body is checked, the EMT-Basic is looking for eight specific symptoms, which can be remembered by the mnemonic DCAP-BTLS (pronounced *deecap-BTLS*). To help remember the mnemonic, remember that **DCAP** means decapitation, and **BTLS** means **Basic Trauma Life Support**. The **DCAP-BTLS** signs are:

- Deformity
- Contusions
- Abrasions
- Punctures
- Burns
- Tenderness
- Lacerations
- Swelling

DCAP-BTLS Sequence

- The head and neck are first evaluated for DCAP-BTLS. In addition, the EMT-Basic at this time also checks the neck for jugular vein distention and/or tracheal shift, either of which would be an indicator of a tension pneumothorax, which would require immediate transport.

- After the assessment of the head and neck, the cervical spine should be secured with a rigid cervical collar. The assessment should then continue with the chest, and in addition to checking for DCAP-BTLS, the EMT-Basic should include the auscultation of breath sounds and signs of paradoxical motion (one area of the chest moving opposite to the others), an indication of a flail segment, which is defined as two or more ribs broken in two or more places.

- The abdomen is then checked for DCAP-BTLS, and all four quadrants are palpated looking for rigidity or tenderness, which may indicate an intra-abdominal bleed and require an expedited transport.

- The pelvis should then be checked for DCAP-BTLS and palpated for stability. The genitals are then checked for wounds, hemorrhage, or discoloration, and, in a male patient, for an erection (priapism), which may indicate a spinal injury.

- The extremities should be checked next, and then the posterior region. If the patient is lying supine, then this examination should be done as he or she is logrolled onto a spine board.

- Baseline vital signs are done at this point and recorded. If the patient is conscious, or if there is a bystander who is familiar with the patient, than a SAMPLE history is taken. The patient is then properly packaged and secured to the board and readied for transport.

Trauma Scores

A trauma score is calculated at this point. A trauma score is a numerical index based on the severity of injury and patient condition. The method of scoring differs from system to system, but most will assign index numbers based on blood pressure, respiratory rate, and the **Glasgow Coma Scale** (GCS). To calculate the Glasgow Coma Scale, assign the following index numbers as appropriate:

- Eye opening: 4 if spontaneous, 3 if to voice, 2 if to pain, 1 if eyes will not open.

- Verbal response: 5 if oriented, 4 if confused, 3 if inappropriate, 2 if incomprehensible, 1 if no response.

- Motor response: 6 if patient obeys commands, 5 if patient localizes pain, 4 if patient withdraws from pain, 3 if patient flexes extremities to pain, 2 if patient extends extremities to pain, 1 if no response.

Thus a patient without any deficiencies would receive a score of 15, while a patient completely unconscious and nonresponsive would receive a score of 3.

The most commonly used **Revised Trauma Score** is calculated as follows:

- Respiratory rate: 10 to 29 breaths per minute equals index number 4, greater than 29 per minute index number 3, 6 to 9 breaths per minute index number 2, 1 to 5 breaths per minute index number 1, if apneic 0.

- Systolic blood pressure: If greater than 89mm, the index number is 4, if between 76 and 88mm the index number is 3, if between 50 and 75mm the index number is 2, if between 1 and 49mm the index number is 1, if there is no pulse or zero blood pressure the index number is 0.

- The Glasgow Coma Scale index: GCS between 13 and 15 the index number is 4, between 9 and 12 the index is 3, between 6 and 8 the index is 2, between 4 and 5 the index is 1, and less than 4 the index is 0.

The maximum revised trauma score therefore would be 12 (4 points for normal respiratory rate, 4 for normal blood pressure, and 4 for a maximum GCS). A patient who is conscious and alert times three, who has fallen from a stepladder, and who presents with abdominal pain which he is guarding with his right hand, has a respiratory rate of 20, and has a blood pressure of 80/60 would be given a revised trauma score of 11. His guarding would lose him a point on the GCS, but would not affect his revised trauma score. The only point lost on the trauma score would be from the low blood pressure.

Once this step is completed, a transport decision is made as to which facility to go to, and transport is begun. While the unit is en route, the EMT-Basic then moves on to the detailed physical exam.

DETAILED PHYSICAL EXAM

The detailed physical exam enables the EMT-Basic to get a clearer picture of the patient's illness or injury and thus gives a more complete picture of what has transpired and is continuing to transpire as the patient is being transported to the emergency room. The purpose of the focused exam was to identify and treat life-threatening conditions and stabilize the patient. Now a more complete exam may reveal conditions that will allow the EMT to assist the physician in making a definitive diagnosis, which can expedite treatment once the patient arrives at the receiving facility.

Exam Procedures

- The DCAP-BTLS mnemonic is used as each section of the body is closely examined both visually and by touch. Each EMT develops a system that enables him or her to perform a complete patient assessment, but almost everyone begins with the crown of the head, inspecting and palpating for signs of DCAP-BTLS, then moving from the top to the posterior neck and coming around to the face, inspecting the ears for signs of fluid, which may indicate a cranial injury.

- The face is then closely examined for trauma and DCAP-BTLS. The eyes are also checked for pupil response, color, and foreign bodies. The normal response is often abbreviated as **PERL**, which stands for **P**upils **E**qual **R**eactive to **L**ight. A diagnostic light is shined into the pupils to observe them constricting and then dilating as the light is moved away. Both pupils should respond the same way, and if there is any other response, it should be noted.

- The nose and mouth are then assessed for DCAP-BTLS, fluid, loose or broken teeth, and foreign odors, which may indicate poisonings, overdoses, or abnormal blood-sugar levels.

- The neck is then assessed for DCAP-BTLS. At this time the EMT-Basic should also recheck for jugular vein distension (JVD) and tracheal shift. Remember that these two signs were also checked during the initial trauma assessment and either would have been an indicator for expedited transport for a possible tension pneumothorax. This condition may not have been present initially, but may have developed subsequent to the initial assessment, which is why it is necessary to perform the detailed physical exam and to continually reevaluate. As the lower neck is palpated, the EMT-Basic should also be checking for subcutaneous emphysema, which will manifest itself as a fine bubbling sensation beneath the skin, indicating air under the skin and an underlying air leakage from the respiratory system secondary to chest trauma or illness.

- The chest is next and is checked for DCAP-BTLS. The ribs are palpated for signs of crepitance, tenderness, or fracture. The EMT-Basic must also observe as the patient breathes and be alert for signs of paradoxical motion, which is when an area of the chest moves in the opposite direction of normal motion. On inspiration, the chest rises as the lungs expand and falls as the patient breathes out. If an area of the chest moves in an opposite way during this process, it is indicative of a flail chest segment, where two or more ribs are broken in two or more places. This flail segment is then splinted in accordance with local protocols.

- As part of the chest examination, the lungs should be auscultated with a stethoscope for breath sounds at four points. Beginning at the closest side to the EMT-Basic, the stethoscope should be placed just below the clavicle at the midpoint and used to listen for normal breath sounds, with any other sounds, such as rhonchi, rales, gurgling, or wheezing, noted. It should also be noted if the breath sounds are diminished or absent. Then the stethoscope should be moved to the same point on the opposite side of the patient. Next return to the side of the patient nearest the EMT and listen at the base of the lung on the midaxillary line and then move to the opposite side. This will enable the EMT-Basic to compare and contrast the volume and sounds from the anterior lung fields in both lungs.

- The EMT-Basic next checks the abdomen for DCAP-BTLS. Remember that the dividing line between the chest and abdomen is the diaphragm and the meeting point of the four abdominal quadrants is the navel. Palpating the abdomen requires the EMT-Basic to use the tips of his or her fingers to feel as she or he gently applies pressure to all four quadrants. In addition to DCAP-BTLS, the EMT-Basic is also checking to see if the abdomen is rigid or soft, as rigidity would be indicative of an intra-abdominal bleed. Also, the EMT-Basic should be palpating for a bounding pulse in the abdomen, which may indicate an abdominal aortic aneurysm, which could be fatal if it ruptured.

- Moving inferior to the pelvis, the pelvis is checked for DCAP-BTLS and is gently flexed and compressed to determine stability. The genitals should also be rechecked for hemorrhaging and for priapism in the male.

- Next all four extremities are checked again for DCAP-BTLS. The EMT-Basic will also want to check distal pulses and capillary refill on all four extremities to determine adequate circulation, as well as sensation and motor function of the hands and feet.

- If the patient has been secured to a backboard, it will be difficult to recheck the posterior, so it is imperative that a thorough assessment be done when the patient is log-rolled and checked during the focused trauma assessment.

- The final step in the detailed assessment is to retake vital signs and note especially any wide divergence from the initial vital signs taken during the focused assessment.

ONGOING ASSESSMENT

Once initial and focused assessments have been completed, if the patient is still in the care of the EMT, then the responsibility for the patient remains with the EMT-Basic. Historically, this is the portion of the call during which the patient's condition can change and not be noticed by the EMT-Basic, often with tragic results. Apnea will sometimes occur without any struggle or outward sign, and if it occurs, the EMT-Basic must be ready to deal with this new medical problem. A patient who is stable one minute could conceivably, and often will, become unstable in the next.

As a general rule, vitals signs should be repeated every five minutes and duly noted on the run report (see the Documentation part of this chapter). In addition, head-to-toe assessment should be repeated anytime the EMT-Basic detects any change in patient condition. If a new complaint or condition arises, then a new focused assessment should be done, especially keeping the new complaint or condition in mind. A new assessment may also be called for if a downgrading trend is noticed, in either vital signs or mental status. As new conditions occur, they must be treated as encountered, just as if they had been discovered on initial or first focused assessment, and the receiving facility must be notified as soon as possible of the new information.

COMMUNICATIONS

Providing Emergency Medical Services is a joint effort involving many people, and the success of the endeavor is predicated upon clear and precise communications between the elements of the EMS system. EMS calls usually begin with a phone call to an emergency dispatcher. This call may be to a dedicated emergency line, a 911 call center, or even a routine phone line. The dispatcher is responsible for accurately taking down the location and nature of the call and, if qualified, giving prearrival instructions. This information may be relayed to a second dispatcher who actually dispatches the nearest appropriate EMS unit, usually by two-way radio, and who is responsible for transmitting the information received by the call taker. The EMS unit will give updates and changes in status back to the dispatcher, such as "en route," "arrive on scene," etc.

Communications Technology

The EMT-Basic is also responsible for notifying the receiving hospital of patient information and in many cases for seeking guidance from a physician as to performing procedures described in the applicable protocols. This task was originally done by two-way radio, but is now often done by cellular telephone.

It goes without saying that clear communication between all personnel involved in the EMS system is paramount. As such, communications equipment should be checked at the beginning of each shift to assure that it will function properly during EMS encounters. Also, the use of backup and redundant systems is necessary so that all elements can communicate with each other as needed, even in the event of a large-scale disaster. In after-action reports from almost all major disasters, the lack of communication between public safety units is mentioned as being highly problematic and significant, so systems must take these issues into account when designing and utilizing communications systems.

While most people do not need a lot of training to use a cell phone, since they are rapidly becoming a staple of modern life, the use of a two-way radio does take some getting used to. It is important to remember when using a two-way radio that many units may be sharing a common frequency, so radio courtesy is very important. If someone transmits while another unit is already transmitting, both conversations may become unintelligible.

There is an old saying in citizens band radio: "Engage brain before engaging radio." It should especially apply to public safety radio. Before you key the radio, know exactly what it is you want to communicate to the party who is receiving the information. Speak slowly and clearly, using proper terminology. You have to release the push-to-talk (PTT) switch to receive, so when finished speaking do so. If your system is using radio repeaters to allow for long range communication, you may have to wait a few seconds before transmitting, which also delays the reception of incoming radio traffic.

Confidentiality

When communicating over public safety radio, you must be aware of the need to maintain patient confidentiality, since radio frequencies are monitored by the general public and the news media. Do not give a patient's name over the radio, nor should you give any identifying information that would enable someone listening to identify your patient.

Codes

Even codes commonly in use vary from location to location, and even from service to service. Confidential information should be passed by more secure transmissions, such as cellular telephones. Dispatch systems that use confidential codes for sensitive calls, such as attempted suicide, sexual assault, etc., should assure that these codes are understood by all those who use them in order to prevent confusion when dealing with these types of calls. The National Incident Management System guidelines currently being promulgated by the Department of Homeland Security strongly discourage the use of codes, since mutual aid units may use different codes, causing problems in communications. Codes also may confuse the recipient of a message if they are not conversant with these particular codes.

Communication with the Receiving Facility

When notifying the receiving facility, identify your unit and whether you are BLS (Basic Life Support) or ALS (Advanced Life Support). Give the patient's age, gender, and chief complaint. This enables the person receiving the information to begin to form a mental picture of your patient, which will be crucial in decisions about triage and summoning needed resources. After the chief complaint, give a brief SAMPLE history, the patient's mental status, vital signs, any other pertinent information from your assessment, any treatments you have performed, the patient's response to these interventions, and finally your estimated time of arrival (ETA).

When you arrive at the receiving facility, the triage nurse may or may not have received your report, so you will tell him or her in person what you have told the person on the radio, and then follow the nurse's directions to discharge your patient to the emergency department's care.

Communicating properly with patients is an art that is developed over time. Some points to bear in mind are that the patient is in distress and his or her answers may be vague or may even deny the reason you have been summoned to the location. Your approach to the patient will depend on the circumstances, but the general rule of talking to and treating others as you would want to be treated in the same situation is always applicable. Speak gently and slowly, making eye contact with your patient. Never allow your expressions to betray disgust, doubt, or despair. Try and maintain a neutral expression. Always be courteous, even if your patient is not. Ask the patient's permission before you touch the patient and explain exactly what you are going to do and why you have to do it.

DOCUMENTATION

The documentation of an emergency medical services encounter is called a prehospital care report (PCR), but is commonly referred to as a run report. The bane of any job is paperwork, and emergency medical services are no exception. Since the EMT is medical profession and the United States is the most litigious country in the world, documentation is a skill that is almost as necessary as good patient care. The general rule of documentation is that if it's not written down, it didn't happen. Your medical report may be subpoenaed for either a criminal or civil action, and an attorney may subpoena you as well to testify as to the events in question. It is common for a civil action to take up to seven years to reach a jury trial, and you may have to recount facts seven years after the occurrence. You may remember inserting an oropharyngeal airway, but if the written report of the event consists solely of "no breathing, started CPR", then the attorney will present to the jury that the OPA was perhaps never inserted.

Good Documentation is Good Patient Care

In addition to the legal considerations, good documentation is also a prerequisite for good patient care. The EMT-Basic is often the first medical provider to interact with a patient, and his or her observations may be critical in the patient's course of treatment. The physician who ultimately becomes responsible for a patient's care may be far removed by both time and distance from the EMT-Basic who began care, and the PCR may be the only way the physician can picture the situation that brought the patient to her care.

For example, you arrive on the scene of a "man down" call. The patient is a forty-year-old male who is actively seizing with his hands clenched and rotated inward. As you reach the patient's side, the seizure subsides, and his hands relax to a normal position and he is now unconscious. There is no indication of trauma, so you perform an initial assessment that is unremarkable and the bystanders are not aware of any medical history. You transport to the nearest emergency room, and en route the patient begins to regain consciousness, but is confused and disoriented. His vitals remain stable, and as you discharge him to the emergency room, he is becoming more lucid. By the time the physician sees him, he may have completely returned to normal, with no memory of the events that brought him to the hospital. The EMT-Basic's PCR in this case is crucial to the patient's treatment, especially if decorticate posturing was noted (hands clenched and rotated inward), a possible indication of spinal damage.

Contents of the Run Report

The run report will contain the following information: the current date, the patient's name and address, gender, date of birth, phone number, reason for the call, medical history, current medications, and known allergies.

The narrative will give the story of the encounter and should paint a picture but will enable the reader to picture what the EMT-Basic saw and experienced, as well as the interactions he or she took in treating and transporting the patient. The narrative will include any findings made during the patient assessments, including baseline vital signs. It should state clearly and definitively the chief complaint. If the patient states something specific, such as "I had too much to drink," it should be put in quotation marks. The use of abbreviations should be governed by local medical usage.

The run report is a confidential medical document and must be treated accordingly. Completed run reports must be secured and not left out where they can be read by those not involved in the patient's care. If a run report is used for training or educational purposes, any information that could identify the patient must be removed.

Since the PCR is a legal document, it should state only the actual facts of a call as the EMT-Basic records them. False statements, such as those used to cover up an omission of protocol steps, may place the EMT-Basic in danger of losing his or her license to practice as well as open the service and the individual EMT-Basic up to increased legal liability, including possible criminal charges. Falsification of the PCR could lead to inappropriate follow-up care being given by the receiving facility, with possible damage to the patient. This should be sufficient to deter any EMT-Basic from falsifying any statements on the run report.

If any error is made on the PCR, any corrections must be noted and signed. This is usually accomplished by placing a horizontal line through the incorrect information and then noting the date and time of the correction with the initials of the report writer.

As noted before, refusal issues are increasingly problematic to the emergency medical service, so the documentation of patient refusals must be especially thorough. An adult patient of sound mind can refuse medical treatment or transport. If the EMT-Basic believes that a specific treatment or transport to the hospital is appropriate, he or she must explain their rationale to the patient; if the patient continues to refuse, than both the explanation and the patient's refusal must be documented. This narrative should note that the patient was told of the possible results of not following the EMT-Basic's recommendations. Once this narrative is completed, the patient should sign the refusal. The patient's signature should be witnessed by an impartial third party, preferably a police officer if one is on scene. If the patient refuses to sign the release, then a disinterested third party should witness that the EMT-Basic explained the procedures and consequences.

In addition to the prehospital care report, the EMT-Basic must also be familiar with the written documents in use by his or her service. These reports will include injury reports for EMS personnel in the line of duty, auto accident reports following incidents involving the EMS vehicle, infectious-disease-exposure reports, and police witness statements if the EMT-Basic has witnessed a criminal act or is the victim of a crime. Any of these reports should be attached to the PCR for the incident during which they occurred, as well as placed in the appropriate personnel and service files.

PRACTICE SET

1. You respond priority to an assist the police call at a domestic violence incident. You arrive on scene and observe two police cars with their lights flashing in the driveway and a woman lying prone on the lawn in front of the residence. You hear gunfire coming from the residence. Your correct course of action is to

    (A) Request additional rescues immediately.

    (B) Rush to the woman down, stabilize her cervical spine, and check her airway.

    (C) Withdraw your unit from the residence.

    (D) Enter the dwelling to check for additional victims while your partner assists the woman down in the yard.

2. You respond to a fight in progress. The police advise the scene is secure, and you are wearing suitable protective equipment. Your patient is a male, thirtyish, seated on the steps of a residence, bent over and clutching his chest. He is making noisy respiratory sounds and is groaning in pain. You can smell the odor of alcohol. You check his carotid pulse, and he has a good pulse with a rate of 80. There are no signs of gross hemorrhage. Your next step is to perform which of the following assessments?

    (A) Focused medical assessment

    (B) Focused trauma assessment

    (C) Initial assessment

    (D) Medical insurance assessment

3. You are dispatched to a motorcycle accident on the freeway. You respond priority and arrive on scene. You observe three police cars on scene, a destroyed motorcycle lying on its side, and a man lying supine next to the motorcycle with a large piece of the front fork of the motorcycle sticking out of his abdomen. The scene is safe and you are wearing suitable protection. You approach the patient and the next thing you do is

    (A) Check his airway.

    (B) Stabilize the large piece of metal with cravats and bandages.

    (C) Request a physician to the scene to perform a surgical removal.

    (D) Transfer the patient to a backboard and transport immediately.

4. You arrive on scene to find a patient lying supine on the ground. As you approach the patient, you can hear him breathing and observe his chest rising and falling. The scene is secure, and you are wearing appropriate protective equipment. His eyes are closed, and you shake his shoulder and ask his name. He has no response. You shout at him asking if he's all right, and his eyes open and he groans. You ask him what happened, and he does not appear to understand at all. You rub his sternum, and he yells, "Ow!" Which of the following best describes his level of consciousness?

    (A) Conscious and alert

    (B) Responsive to pain

    (C) Responsive to verbal

    (D) Unresponsive

5. You respond to a residence for a man down, possibly intoxicated, call. You arrive after police have secured the scene, and you are wearing proper protective clothing. You observe a large male lying on the floor next to the couch of the living room. There are no bystanders, and he is breathing and has a carotid pulse. There is no gross hemorrhage, and his capillary refill is approximately five seconds. What condition should you suspect?

   (A) Intoxication

   (B) Circulatory compromise

   (C) Respiratory distress

   (D) Diabetic Ketoacidosis

6. Which of the following patients would be given a priority transport?

   (A) Woman in second-stage labor

   (B) Male with chest pain, normal respirations, and a history of prior heart attacks

   (C) Twelve-year-old girl with difficulty breathing and a history of asthma

   (D) Two-year-old who fell out of his crib and is crying loudly

7. Which of the following patients would be given a priority transport?

   (A) Male patient conscious and alert with a blood pressure of 210/110

   (B) Female patient in labor with respiratory rate of 20 per minute

   (C) Male patient with a pulse rate of 110 per minute

   (D) Female patient with a pulse rate of 20 per minute

8. Who can answer the SAMPLE questions for a patient assessment?

   (A) Police

   (B) Bystanders

   (C) Your partner

   (D) The patient

9. Which of the following conditions noted during the focused trauma assessment would indicate immediate transport?

   (A) Unconscious

   (B) Low blood sugar

   (C) Tracheal shift to right

   (D) Pedestrian struck by car on city street

10. You are dispatched for a bicyclist struck by a car. On your arrival, your patient is lying supine on the ground, not moving. You approach your patient from the feet, take manual stabilization of his head, and check his airway. He is breathing and you can palpate a carotid pulse, which appears rapid. You ask in a loud voice if he is okay and get no response. Your partner rubs the patient's sternum with his thumb and your patient opens his eyes, groans, and moves his hand to his chest to push your partner's hand away. There is a large bruise with swelling on the right side of his head and no other apparent injuries. His vital signs are BP 160/100, pulse 60, respirations 15. What do you calculate his revised trauma score to be?

    (A) 8

    (B) 9

    (C) 10

    (D) 11

11. You arrive on the scene of an MVA, car vs. pole. Your patient is a twenty-five-year-old female who was ejected from her vehicle when it struck the telephone pole. The car is totally demolished. Your initial assessment is that your patient is unconscious and nonresponsive. Due to the severity of the car's damage, you determine that this is a "load and go," package your patient, and begin transport. As you do your focused trauma assessment, you notice that the patient's left upper quadrant is now rigid, whereas in the initial assessment it appeared normal. What should be your next action?

    (A) Continue your focused trauma assessment, having noted the rigidity.

    (B) Start an IV 0.9 percent NaCl WO.

    (C) Request your driver to expedite as you suspect your patient has an intra-abdominal bleed.

    (D) Perform a modified jaw thrust.

12. You are dispatched to a report of a female intoxicated. The scene is secure and you are wearing suitable precautions. You arrive on scene and find a female in her forties lying supine, unconscious and responsive (groans) to painful stimuli. You detect an odor of alcohol and her friend confirms that she has been drinking vodka shots heavily all evening. There is no indication of trauma and your initial assessment is unremarkable. You place the patient in the truck, administer 10 liters oxygen via nonrebreather mask and begin priority transport to the nearest emergency room, 15 minutes away. You notify the hospital of the patient's condition and vital signs. After disconnecting from the hospital, you begin to reassess your patient and now notice that she is not breathing. Your next step is to

    (A) Advise the driver to expedite.

    (B) Insert an oropharyngeal airway and ventilate at 12–15 times per minute.

    (C) Continue the assessment to try and discover any other conditions.

    (D) Retake pulse, respiratory rate, and blood pressure.

13. When you are giving information to the receiving facility, which of the following should not be given over the radio?

    (A) Patient's vital signs

    (B) Patient's level of consciousness

    (C) Patient's name

    (D) Estimated time of arrival

14. Which of the following calls should NOT be responded to as a priority (lights and siren) response?

    (A) Difficulty breathing

    (B) Chest pain

    (C) Motor vehicle accident

    (D) Possible ankle sprain

15. Which of the following statements about a dispatch call are true?

    (A) The dispatcher will tell you exactly what you will find when you arrive on scene.

    (B) The dispatcher is familiar with all aspects of the call and will relay them to you.

    (C) The dispatcher will tell you what information he or she has, but it may be incomplete.

    (D) The dispatcher's information is completely unreliable.

16. You are radio-dispatched to a "Code C" nonpriority. You have no idea what a "Code C" is, and when you look at your partner he shrugs his shoulders. Your next step should be to

    (A) Respond and try to figure it out.

    (B) Key the radio and ask the dispatcher to tell you what a "Code C" is in English.

    (C) Call the dispatcher on the cell phone and ask him or her to explain to you what a "Code C" is.

    (D) Respond priority even though you don't know what "Code C" is.

17. As you are writing the narrative portion of the PCR following an automobile accident, you write that the patient's left pupil was fixed and dilated and the right was PERL. Your partner says, "Wasn't the right pupil fixed and dilated?" You realize that you wrote the wrong eye in the narrative. Which of the following is the correct next step?

    (A) Rip the run report into small pieces and dispose of it in the shredder.

    (B) Forget about it.

    (C) Write a new report and staple it to the incorrect report.

    (D) Draw a line through the word "left" and write above it "right" with the date, time, and your initials, and note that you corrected the report at the bottom of the narrative.

18. You arrive on the scene of a one-car motor vehicle accident. The car left the lane of travel and struck the soft shoulder, where it appears to have rolled over at least once. The driver is a female, approximate age 40, who is conscious, alert, and oriented times three. Your partner applies head stabilization from the backseat while you conduct the assessment. The patient states that she's fine and just wants a ride to the hospital. The windshield is cracked and the patient is not wearing a seat belt. She has a bruise on the front of her forehead. You explain that you want to apply a cervical collar and then a Kendrick Extrication Device (KED) to remove her from the vehicle to protect her spine. She becomes agitated and announces that all she wants is a ride to the hospital and that she doesn't want you to do anything other than that. She begins to get out of the car. Which of the following statements is correct?

    (A) The best course of action at this time is to let her walk herself to the truck and transport her to the hospital.

    (B) Notify her that the police will place her in protective custody and then you will be able to do whatever you want.

    (C) Explain to her the risks of spinal injury unless you take the proper precautions and, if she continues to refuse, fill out a narrative documenting your explanation and her refusal and have her sign it in the presence of the police.

    (D) Disregard her protests and apply the cervical collar and KED.

19. You respond to a call to the police station for a male with chest pains. You respond priority with appropriate BSI precautions. You arrive on scene and find a male in his forties seated in a chair clutching his chest, in obvious distress. He is pale, diaphoretic, and having difficulty breathing. There is no indication of trauma. He states that he's fine and refuses all treatment and transport options. He is not in police custody, but is the victim of a crime. Which of the following options is most appropriate?

    (A) Explain the consequences of his refusal and have him sign the refusal form and have it witnessed by a police officer.

    (B) Disregard his objections, administer oxygen via nonrebreather, and transport priority to the nearest hospital emergency room.

    (C) Patiently explain to the patient the seriousness of his condition and continue to encourage him to allow you to treat him and transport him to the hospital.

    (D) When his eyes are closed, administer 1/150 NTG sublingual.

20. The patient in question 19 becomes unconscious as you are trying to get him to agree to go to the hospital. He has never given you permission for treatment or transport, so your next move would be to

    (A) Initiate appropriate treatment under the doctrine of implied consent.

    (B) Document that the patient never gave permission to treat, note that the patient is now unconscious and cannot sign the refusal, and have a police officer sign verifying your explanation.

    (C) Transport the patient priority, but do not perform any treatments since you do not have the patient's permission.

    (D) Initiate appropriate treatment in accordance with local protocols under the doctrine of expressed consent.

ANSWER EXPLANATIONS

1. C

The scene is not safe and you should not be there. You can request additional rescues (A) at any time. Your primary inclination may be to run to the woman (B), but you run the risk of becoming a victim yourself. Entering a dwelling from which you hear gunfire (D) is incredibly dangerous and will most likely result in you being shot.

2. C

The temptation is to answer (B), as this is most probably a trauma, but taking shortcuts compromises the EMT-Basic's ability to make the correct determinations. The EMT-Basic's ability to develop good practice skills will be governed by a willingness to follow protocols; if the EMT-Basic develops this skill early, then he or she will develop into an excellent practitioner.

3. A

Even though this is a "load and go" situation due to the magnitude of the patient's injuries, a patient without an airway will arrive at the ER dead. If the patient has a patent airway, is breathing, and has a pulse, then stabilize the metal (B) and prepare for immediate transport. Requesting a physician to the scene (C) would take too much time and would endanger the patient more. The metal can be removed best in an operating room.

4. C

He did not respond to normal stimuli so he is not conscious and alert. The next level is verbal and this is where he responded. He also responded to pain, but the higher level (verbal) would apply. Since he did respond to both verbal and pain, he is not unresponsive.

5. B

This is a challenging question and the quick answer without performing a complete assessment is (D). In rereading the question, other than the dispatch, there are no indicators in your primary assessment that indicate alcohol. The fact that his nail beds take so long to return to pink would indicate that his circulation is impaired, and although respiratory compromise and DKA are possibilities, circulation is the better answer.

6. C

While all the choices here are possibilities if secondary assessments find something significant or conditions change, the patient with difficulty breathing needs to be expedited.

7. D

A patient with a pulse of 20 will present with symptoms of low perfusion including pale skin and diminished level of consciousness. The other vital signs may be out of normal range, but in the absence of a life-threatening condition would be considered nonpriority transport.

8. D

SAMPLE stands for the section of the medical assessment that enables you to get a better idea of the patient's chief complaint. It stands for Signs and symptoms, Allergies, Medications, Past medical history, Last oral intake, and Events leading up to this situation. Bystanders may be able to give you some of the events, but the patient is the source for most of this information. A SAMPLE history becomes more problematic when the patient is unconscious or incoherent. Family members may be able to fill in some of the SAMPLE history as well.

9. C

Tracheal shift to either side is indicative of a tension pneumothorax, a collapsed lung that is pushing against other organs and may lead to other organ failure or damage. It can be relieved only by a chest tube, which is beyond the scope of the EMT-Basic. (A) is a condition that should have been found in the initial assessment and by itself does not indicate immediate transport. Neither does low blood sugar, which can be treated by the EMT-Basic in the field. A pedestrian struck has a high incidence of suspicion due to the nature of injury, but, again, by itself is not indicative of an immediate transport.

10. D

The first thing you must calculate is the Glasgow Coma Scale. His eyes open to pain, giving him a 2, his words are incomprehensible, giving him a 2, and he localizes pain, which gives him a 5. Therefore, the total GCS is 9, making the trauma score index a 3. In calculating the trauma score, he gets 4 for respiratory rate between 10 and 29, 4 for having a systolic blood pressure greater than 89, and 3 for the GCS, which gives him a trauma score of 11. Use care in calculating mathematical questions like this one, since one of your choices is 9, which is the GCS. It's always a good idea to run calculations twice to be sure.

11. C

While you suspected a serious injury before, the development of a rigid left upper quadrant is fairly indicative of a ruptured spleen, which will result in the patient's bleeding intra-abdominally. The only treatment for this condition is removal of the spleen in an operating room. You may continue the assessment to look for further conditions, or request an ALS intercept for the IV, but both of these will be dependent on the time constraint. Remember, your goal is get this patient to an operating room as soon as possible, so your actions should lend themselves to that result. The modified jaw thrust should have already been done on the scene, not at this time.

12. B

A patient needs oxygen to live, and if she is not breathing, then she will die. The airway must first be secured and then the patient ventilated. You can advise the driver to expedite once this is taken care of. (C) and (D) can be undertaken if you have another EMT in the back of the truck, but if you are alone, your concern must be for the patient's airway and respirations.

13. C

To protect your patient's confidentiality, you will almost never give a patient's name over the radio; however, all of the other answers are important to the triage and preparation for treating your patient.

14. D

The first three answers all call for a priority response. In the absence of other information, the response to a simple non-life-threatening condition, such as a sprained ankle, should be non-priority.

15. C

The correct answer is (C). A good dispatcher will relay the proper information to you, but what he or she has received from the calling party may be incomplete. The dispatcher is only relaying to you the information the caller has given, and the caller may not have a complete picture either, so what you find may be completely different. However, the dispatcher is giving you the best assessment available at the time, which will contain information that you will need to properly assess the scene, so there is some reliability, but always take what you're told with a grain of salt.

16. C

The correct answer is (C) because it is private. (B) is an incorrect answer since it now broadcasts to anyone listening what a "Code C" is and negates further the value of using codes. (A) and (D) can be ruled out because they are the same answer and a bad way for an EMT-Basic to work as well.

17. D

Since most jurisdictions serialize their reports, ripping up the narrative sheet will put the sequence out of order. Destroying a written run report also casts suspicion upon the reason it was done; it may be perceived as destroying evidence in a criminal or civil matter. The fact that one particular eye was fixed and dilated and the other was not is material to the patient's condition and will impact the subsequent treatment, so it must be corrected and noted and cannot simply be ignored. Two reports would confuse the issue as to which report was correct, so (C) is also inappropriate.

18. C

(C) describes the appropriate course of action in this matter. (A) is wrong because you have not yet documented your explanation and treatment options, and if she persists, you may become liable for injuries. (B) is wrong because unless the police have probable cause for placing the person in protective custody, they will not do it. (D) may be considered assault and battery.

19. C

The potential seriousness of the situation really requires you to stand by as long as possible. (A) is legally correct, but if the patient's condition changes as soon as you drive out of the parking lot, a jury might consider it abandonment. (B) is assault and battery, and possibly kidnapping. (D) is also assault, since you do not have the patient's permission to give treatment, even if it is allowed by your protocols.

20. A

Implied consent means that an unconscious patient would want you to treat him if he were conscious, even if he initially declined. This doctrine is well established in case law. (B) is abandonment, (C) is as well, and (D) is incorrect because expressed consent would be the patient's agreeing to your treatment and transport recommendations, which this patient never did.

Chapter Six: **Medical Emergencies**

- Pharmacology

- Respiratory Emergencies

- Cardiovascular Emergencies

- Diabetes

- Seizures

- Allergies

- Poisoning and Overdose

- Environmental Emergencies

- Behavioral Emergencies

- Obstetric and Gynecological Emergencies

In the practice of prehospital emergency medicine, the EMT-Basic, dependent upon local protocols, may be instructed to administer various medications. It is important that the EMT-Basic understand what these medications are, how they work, for what medical conditions they are administered (indications), and under which circumstances they should not be administered (contraindications). The EMT-Basic must always be guided by the local protocols as to drug administration since, these protocols vary widely from locale to locale.

PHARMACOLOGY

The following four medications are carried on almost all EMT-Basic units in the United States: oxygen, oral glucose, activated charcoal, and aspirin. Their use and dosages will be covered in the chapters of this book for the specific conditions for which they are indicated. In addition, many EMS systems now allow EMT-Basics to administer medications that are already prescribed for a particular patient. These drugs may include asthma medications administered by metered dose inhaler such as albuterol, metaproterenol, and ipratropium; nitroglycerin prescribed for angina; and epinephrine for treatment of anaphylaxis.

Medications may be administered to the patient in a variety of ways. These include: injection, both intramuscular and subcutaneous; inhalation; oral; sublingual; and rectal. In order to accommodate the various routes of administration, medications also come in a variety of forms, including compressed pills or tablets, liquid gels, suspensions, aerosols, gases, sprays, and suppositories. Individual protocols will indicate which medications may be given under which circumstances, which circumstances will preclude their administration, the route of administration, and the dosage.

The Five Rights

When administering pharmaceuticals, the EMT-Basic must be aware of the "Five Rights" involved in drug therapy. If a specific protocol allows the administration of a drug and medical control concurs, the EMT-Basic is responsible for verifying the following: Right Medication, Right Patient, Right Route, Right Dose, and Right Date.

When medication is administered, the date and time should be noted and then documented in the run report. Following drug administration, as with any treatment, the patient should always be reassessed to see if there are any changes in the patient's condition, including vital signs.

EMT-Basics would do well to become familiar with the more common prescription medications, as they can be clues to potential problems. Two good references to have on hand are the *Physician's Desk Reference®* (*PDR*), which lists almost all medications currently in use in the United States, their chemical composition, indications, and contraindications as well as other useful information. Another good source is *ePocrates®*, a software program that can be downloaded into the EMT-Basic's personal data assistant. The program is not as comprehensive as the PDR, but is good for recognizing medical conditions for which a particular medication is being prescribed.

RESPIRATORY EMERGENCIES

One of the most common EMS dispatches is for difficulty breathing, or dyspnea. The causes and manifestations of this broad-based condition include asthma, bronchitis, and emphysema. The severity of respiratory emergencies can range from simple dyspnea to apnea, or cessation of respiratory function. (This is a good time to review the anatomy and physiology of the respiratory system, which is necessary to recognize and treat the various conditions that come under this heading.)

The signs and symptoms of dyspnea may include any of the following: shortness of breath (SOB), restlessness, increased pulse rate, changes in respiratory rate (>20 or <12), changes in skin color (bluish gray, pale, or flushed), noisy respirations (crowing, wheezing, gurgling, snoring, or stridor), inability to speak, use of accessory muscles to breathe, altered mental status, abdominal breathing, coughing, irregular breathing rhythm, patient in tripod position (hunched forward with arms rotated outward), and barrel chest.

Emergency Care of Dyspnea

If the patient is conscious and able to answer questions, the OPQRST (Onset, Provocation, Quality, Radiation, Severity, Time of onset) questions are appropriate at this time. These are then followed by the SAMPLE (Signs and symptoms, Allergies, Medications, Past history, Last oral intake, and Events leading to this condition) questions. In addition to these questions, if the patient indicates that he or she has an inhaler or uses some other intervention, then you want to ask if the patient has used one of these interventions since the onset of this set of symptoms and whether or not there was any change in his or her condition as a result. If the patient is unconscious or unable to speak, than a family member may have to be the source for this information.

If the complaint is dyspnea, then vital signs are taken at this point, including a baseline pulse oximeter reading. Depending on the patient's signs, symptoms, and oxygen saturation reading, the EMT-Basic may then apply oxygen via the appropriate device in accordance with local protocol. Auscultation of the chest would be next, listening in the six fields for noises and normal or diminished breath sounds. If the patient has an inhaler, or your protocols allow you to administer a breathing treatment, you may then contact medical control with the information and request a consultation and orders for the appropriate intervention. As the treatment is being given, you then complete the focused assessment and begin preparations for transport.

It is important to note at this point that continued assessment is critical, as many times dyspnea may be a prelude to a more serious airway condition and the EMT-Basic must be prepared to intervene as appropriate, including the use of airway adjuncts and ventilation as per his or her level of training, and the applicable protocols.

Bronchodilators

Since most states allow the administration of bronchodilators by EMT-Basics, the EMT-Basic must be familiar with these medications and the methods by which they are administered. Most states will allow, with medical control, the assistance of the EMT-Basic in administering the patient's own prescribed inhaler. The inhaler may be the delivery device for medications such as albuterol, isotharine, and metaproterenol, among others. The trade names for these medications include Proventil™, Ventolin™, Bronkowol™, Alupent™, and Metaprel™. Medications such as Ventolin™ and Proventil™ are beta agonist bronchodilators, which quickly and effectively dilate the bronchioles, reducing airway resistance and allowing air to pass more easily and quickly into the alveoli of the lungs.

Indications for administration of a prescribed inhaler must include all of the following three criteria: 1. The patient must have the signs and symptoms of a respiratory emergency. 2. The patient's physician must have prescribed the inhaler. and 3. The EMT-Basic must have authority from the medical control. If any of these conditions are not met, then the use of the inhaler is contraindicated. Also, if the patient has used the inhaler prior to the arrival of EMS, the number of times and amounts administered must be relayed to the medical control, as the patient may have reached or exceeded the maximum dose for that particular medication.

If medical control gives the order for administration of a handheld metered dose inhaler, the EMT-Basic then verifies the five Rights (Medication, Patient, Route, Dose, and Date). The EMT-Basic then should shake the inhaler vigorously several times and assure that the inhaler is at room temperature. The EMT-Basic then removes any oxygen adjuncts from the patient and asks the patient to exhale deeply, then has the patient place his or her lips around the mouthpiece of the device, depressing the container as he or she inhales deeply. The patient should hold his or her breath for as long as possible in order to allow the medication to be absorbed into the tissues of the lungs. Finally, the EMT-Basic should replace the oxygen adjunct and reassess the patient. Remember that a patient with a prescribed inhaler will usually have received detailed instructions on its use and may not need all of these details. Be aware of the possible side effects of these medications, including tachycardia, tremors, and increased anxiety, and be prepared to manage these if and when they occur.

Conditions That May Lead to Dyspnea

The EMT-Basic must be familiar with the various diseases and conditions that may lead to dyspnea. These include emphysema and chronic bronchitis, which are lumped together under the generic name of chronic obstructive pulmonary disease (COPD). Other diseases that may cause dyspnea are: asthma, pneumonia, pulmonary embolism, pulmonary edema (many times secondary to congestive heart failure), spontaneous pneumothorax, and hyperventilation syndrome.

CARDIOVASCULAR EMERGENCIES

Closely following difficulty breathing in the frequency of emergency medical calls is the call for chest pains and possible heart attack. The EMT-Basic must be quick to summon an Advanced Life Support (ALS) intercept and assist for these types of calls, but since the EMT-Basic is most often the first medical provider on the scene, he or she must be confident in his or her ability to perform Basic Life Support (BLS), which may be the defining treatment intervention in patient survival. The American Heart Association™ Chain of Survival studies have shown that the survivability of a sudden cardiac arrest increases dramatically with early access (911), early CPR, early defibrillation, and early Advanced Cardiac Life Support (ACLS). The AHA is quick to point out that ACLS is a follow up to BLS and does not replace it; therefore the EMT-Basic as a BLS provider is an important link in this chain of survival.

A quick review of the anatomy of the cardiovascular system reminds us that the heart is a specialized muscle with a unique electrical system that causes the pumping action of the heart. It is the failure or malfunctioning of this electrical system that brings on the signs and symptoms of a heart attack (myocardial infarction). It is also a mechanical system subject to blockages and mechanical failure. The EMT-Basic should be familiar with the major anatomical points for palpating a pulse. These include the radius at the wrist, the brachia in the upper arm, the posterior tibial and dorsalis pedal in the feet, the carotid in the neck, and the femoral in the upper leg. The pressure in millimeters of mercury as the ventricles contract and send this pulse through the arteries is called the systolic pressure and the pressure when the ventricles are dilating is called the diastolic.

If circulation is inadequate, as may be caused by a loss of fluid from a traumatic injury or from inadequate pumping action of the heart, this is called shock, or hypoperfusion syndrome. The signs and symptoms of shock include: pale or cyanotic skin color, cool clammy skin, weak rapid pulse, rapid shallow breathing, anxiety, altered mental status, nausea and vomiting, low or decreasing blood pressure, and low body temperature.

These signs and symptoms may be present in a trauma victim, which would lead the EMT-Basic to expect significant blood loss from an internal or external injury. If, however, the patient has not been subjected to trauma, and these signs coexist with signs and symptoms of cardiac compromise, such as chest pain or pressure, sudden onset of sweating, difficulty breathing, a feeling of impending doom, and irregular pulse, then the EMT-Basic should suspect that the patient's heart has possibly been affected by some type of electrical or mechanical obstruction.

Emergency Care of Cardiac Compromise

It is beyond the scope of Basic Life Support to diagnose and treat specific cardiac conditions. Consequently, the EMT-Basic must be alert that this is an Advanced Life Support situation and requires either an ALS intercept or rapid transport to an emergency room. With the patient's best interests in mind, the EMT-Basic must make a decision which of these two options to execute, based upon the time each will require. If there is a blockage of a coronary artery, then the portion of the heart that vessel feeds is being deprived of oxygen and is becoming ischemic (dying). The longer definitive treatment, either medical or surgical, is delayed, the larger the area of ischemia and the more damage done.

Emergency care of the suspected cardiac compromise falls into two categories. If a pulse is absent, then the indicated treatment is possible defibrillation with an AED (see following section) and CPR (cardiopulmonary resuscitation). If the suspected cardiac patient has a pulse, then the EMT-Basic should move on to the initial assessment, focused history, and physical exam. In a patient with chest pain and dyspnea who is lying on his or her back, many times relief is obtained simply by sitting the patient up into a Fowler (seated) or semi-Fowler (45-degree angle) position. With a conscious patient, the EMT-Basic should be guided by what the patient says as to which position is most comfortable.

In the typical cardiac scenario with symptoms of chest pain or pressure, dyspnea, cyanotic color, and anxiety, obtain baseline vital signs, including pulse oximetry, and then apply oxygen in the highest concentration tolerated. The OPQRST series of questions is important in the proper assessment of chest pain and will be communicated to the emergency room so that personnel there may properly triage the patient. Especially important is the description of the quality of the pain and whether it is stationary or radiating. Remember that time is tissue in a heart attack (myocardial infarction). If the EMT-Basic performs an adequate focused exam and relays a complete picture to the triage nurse, then time is saved at the triage desk, and the patient is processed quickly to a more definitive level of care that may minimize the damage to his or her heart.

Medications for Cardiac Care

Current studies have shown that aspirin, taken daily as a prophylactic, or given at the onset of chest pain, dramatically improves a patient's chances of survival. Consequently, many local protocols now call for the EMT-Basic to administer aspirin to chest-pain patients, providing they have not already taken one.

Many times the patient has already had a prior episode and may have been prescribed nitroglycerin (NTG) tablets to treat sudden onset chest pain. If your local protocol allows you to administer NTG, or assist the patient in administering it, check with your medical control and follow all directions. NTG is a powerful vasodilator that is placed beneath the patient's tongue (sublingually) and is rapidly absorbed, causing the arteries to dilate. NTG also comes in a spray that is applied sublingually. Side effects may include a drop in blood pressure and headache. If the chest pain is alleviated with NTG, then the physician may suspect that the cause of the chest pain is not myocardial infarction, but a spasm in the coronary arteries called angina pectoris. It is important to be sure that the patient's systolic blood pressure is higher than 100mm when giving NTG, since a drop in blood pressure may result in hypoxia. It's also important to continue retaking blood pressure once you have administered NTG to monitor the effect of the drug.

CPR and Automated External Defibrillators (AED)

Remember that while not every chest-pain patient is going to lapse into cardiac arrest, it can and does happen. Continued assessment is important in these cases. If the patient does suddenly go into cardiac arrest, the EMT-Basic must be prepared to respond immediately. With any chest-pain patient, it is always good to be prepared for this possibility by having the devices you will need to intervene with CPR ready and available. These will include the AED (automated external defibrillator), a bag-valve mask, OPAs, and suctioning equipment.

The EMT-Basic is required by almost all jurisdictions to be current in Healthcare Provider CPR by the American Heart Association™ or Professional Rescuer CPR by the American Red Cross™. These courses now include training in automated external defibrillators (AED). These can be found in public places and may be used by those trained in their use. An AED is a computer-driven device that analyzes a patient's cardiac rhythm and determines whether a countershock is advised. The purpose of this countershock is to reestablish a perfusing rhythm. Current research indicates that if the patient's heart is in either ventricular tachycardia or ventricular fibrillation, a shock delivered as soon as possible after either of these conditions occurs may convert these irregular rhythms to a rhythm that will once again generate a pulse.

The AED does not take the place of CPR, but is an adjunct to it. The correct sequence of use of the AED and CPR is as follows:

1. Determine if the scene is safe and that appropriate infection control precautions are in place.
2. Perform initial assessment, stop CPR if in progress, and verify that the patient has no pulse and is not breathing.
3. Have your partner continue CPR while you prepare and attach the AED.
4. Stop CPR and push the AED "analyze" button. Follow the directions on the machine as to whether or not to shock. Be sure that all personnel are clear of the patient when the AED is analyzing and shocking the patient.

5. Following the shock or the indication that no shock is advised, check for pulse and resume CPR if pulse is absent.

6. Following use of the AED, prepare the patient for transport if the transport time to the emergency room is less than the time it would take for an ALS unit to arrive.

7. If ALS is delayed, then transport the patient once a pulse is restored, six shocks have been delivered, or the AED gives three consecutive messages (after one minute of CPR) that no shock is advised.

8. If the AED has restored the pulse and you are en route, check the patient continually for a pulse. If the pulse disappears, have the driver stop the vehicle and repeat the CPR-AED protocol.

DIABETES

Diabetes mellitus (DM) is a disease of the endocrine system that inhibits the body's ability to metabolize sugar. It will result in a condition known as hyperglycemia, or high blood sugar, and is treated by injections of synthetic insulin, which are usually taken one or more times per day. The condition of a patient on a regular regimen of insulin is called insulin-dependent diabetes mellitus, or IDDM.

Hypoglycemia

Emergency medical services will get involved with IDDM patients when they begin to exhibit symptoms of altered mental status brought on by hypoglycemia or low blood sugar. This is most often caused by taking the prescribed dosage of insulin and not following up with the regular ingestion of food as prescribed, causing the blood sugar to drop. In addition to missing a meal, vomiting, unusual exercise, and ingestion of alcohol are all events that can cause blood sugar to drop and cause the patient to either behave strangely or suddenly become unconscious. The patient's breath at these times may have a fruity odor.

Altered Mental Status

Even though diabetes is paired with altered mental status in many EMT-Basic curricula and most protocols, it is important not to assume that everyone who exhibits signs and symptoms of altered mental status has diabetes, hyperglycemia, or hypoglycemia. Altered mental status may be the result of many other causes, including cerebral hemorrhage, trauma, drug overdose, and disease processes, topics we will discuss later in this chapter.

Persons with IDDM most often will wear Medic Alert™ bracelets that identify them as having this condition, so that when they are found unconscious or impaired, the first presumption is that this is a condition of hypoglycemia, especially if the signs and symptoms develop after missing a meal, vomiting a meal, unusual exercise, or physical activity. The person affected may exhibit symptoms of intoxication, including staggered gait, slurred speech, and being unresponsive to verbal commands. In addition, the heart rate is usually accelerated and the skin will be cool and clammy to the touch. The patient may be completely unconscious and unresponsive or may have a seizure. Many times the patient will present as anxious and combative.

Glucose and Glucagon

Most state protocols will allow EMT-Basics to administer oral glucose to patients who present with these symptoms and are conscious. If the condition is the result of hypoglycemia, the patient will usually respond very quickly to the oral sugar. Some states will allow EMT-Basics to administer glucagon via intramuscular injection. Glucagon is a protein that causes sugar stored in the liver to be released into the bloodstream (and consequently is ineffective in patients with chronic liver disease, such as cirrhosis or hepatitis).

In addition, many states now allow basic EMS units to carry portable glucometers that enable the EMT-Basic to accurately gauge the blood sugar level. This may be especially important to the treating physician, as it will give a baseline blood sugar reading prior to any intervention by EMS. The normal range of blood sugar is 80 to 120 mg/dl, although the range in patients with chronic diabetes may be much wider before physical symptoms occur.

SEIZURES

Seizures, or involuntary muscular activity, may be caused by hypoglycemia, head injuries, and brain diseases such as epilepsy. Prolonged seizures are a true medical emergency, since patients in this condition will begin to develop a lack of oxygen to the brain that could result in brain damage or brain death.

Most seizures are of short duration, and the active portion of the seizure has usually subsided when EMS arrives on the scene. Seizures are followed by a period of unconsciousness or semi-consciousness referred to as the postictal phase. In the pediatric population, seizures are often the result of high body temperatures. These seizures are referred to as febrile seizures.

Treatment of the seizure patient who is in the postictal phase follows the usual pattern of assuring a patent airway and transporting the patient on his or her side (recumbent) in the event of vomiting. If the EMT-Basic cannot rule out the possibility of trauma, then the patient is secured with a cervical collar, head blocks, and a spine board to guard against spinal cord injury. The patient is then transported supine and the entire board rolled in the event of vomiting. Remember that seizures may be caused by head trauma.

ALLERGIES

An allergic reaction is an exaggerated immune-system response by the body to a substance. The most common substances that cause allergies are: insect bites and stings; various foods, but predominantly nuts and shellfish; medications; and certain plants. However, any substance may be an allergen, depending on the body's response to it.

Anaphylaxis (Allergic Reactions)

The EMT-Basic should suspect a possible allergic reaction or anaphylaxis, if the patient reports tingling and heat in the face, mouth, or extremities, severe itching, visible hives, flushed skin, and swelling to the extremities. The main concern is to ensure that the airway does not swell shut and prevent the patient from breathing; therefore, dispatches to possible allergic reactions are always treated as priority calls.

Other symptoms of anaphylaxis may include chest tightness and pressure, prolonged uncontrolled coughing, tachypnea, dyspnea, hoarseness, stridor, and audible wheezing. In addition, the pulse rate will be rapid and the blood pressure will be lower as the body attempts to regulate its response to the allergen.

If the reactions include altered mental status, then hypoxia and hypoperfusion may be severe, and immediate treatment is indicated. After the EMT-Basic performs an initial assessment and treats any conditions discovered there, he or she should proceed on to the focused assessment. There the EMT-Basic must be alert to any history of past allergic reactions, the events that immediately preceded the symptoms that prompted the call to the EMS system, and whether those events were related to past allergic reactions. Food allergies may be particularly insidious in this regard. For example, a person with a severe allergy to nuts will avoid nuts, but nut by-products may be used in processing of other foods, and may cause a surprise reaction.

Epinephrine Syringes

As with any medical assessment, following a complete focused assessment, baseline vital signs are obtained and oxygen is administered. Many patients with severe reactions carry preloaded automatic epinephrine syringes (EpiPens™) that deliver 0.3 mg of 1:1000 epinephrine for adults and 0.15 mg for pediatric patients. If the patient has been instructed in its use, the EMT-Basic may assist in administering this device. Caution is urged here, since improper use of such devices may cause injury to the patient or the EMT-Basic.

In some jurisdictions, EMT-Basics, after consulting medical control, can administer the epinephrine syringe to a patient. Epinephrine will reverse the effects of severe anaphylaxis long enough for the patient to be transported to a medical facility for treatment. The effect of epinephrine is to dilate the bronchioles to relieve difficulty breathing, as it constricts the blood vessels and increases the heart rate to help raise the blood pressure and combat hypoperfusion syndrome. As with the administration of all drugs, the EMT-Basic must check the "Five Rights" before administering or assisting with the administration of epinephrine.

After the administration of any medication, it is important to reassess the patient and note especially any changes in the patient's condition. If the patient was having difficulty breathing and had airway swelling that has responded to the epinephrine, then the assessment of anaphylaxis is usually confirmed and the intervention considered timely. Be sure to advise the receiving facility of the outcome of your intervention. As stated before, it is important for the EMT-Basic to recognize that anaphylaxis often begins as dyspnea and that airway management is the most important condition to be managed.

POISONING AND OVERDOSE

A poison is defined as any substance that produces harmful physiological or psychological effects to the body. According to the National Safety Council, poisoning is responsible for approximately 10 percent of all emergency room admissions in the United States. Overdose is when serious physiological and psychological effects occur from the overuse or misuse of any substance by exceeding safe dosages. The substance may be a legal substance, such as alcohol, or an illegal substance, such as cocaine.

The stereotypical poisoning case is that of the child who gets into the cleaning supplies beneath the sink, a relatively infrequent EMS dispatch. In reality, most EMTs deal with a large number of calls involving either alcohol overdose or the use of illegal drugs. Most college EMS units report that 20 to 30 percent of their calls involve alcohol and substance abuse.

Poisons may enter the body in a variety of ways: ingestion, inhalation, injection, and absorption. Ingestion is when the substance is taken by mouth, such as drinking a toxic substance or taking pills. Inhalation occurs when the substance is inhaled into the lungs, such as breathing in poisons like carbon monoxide from car exhaust in a closed space, or snorting cocaine. Injection involves placing the substance directly into the bloodstream using a hypodermic syringe, as with injecting heroin. Absorption occurs when toxins enter the body by contact with the skin, such as with poison ivy or pesticide poisoning.

Signs and symptoms of poisoning will vary depending on the poison and how the body reacts to it. The EMT-Basic must be prepared to intervene if there is a sudden change in the patient's condition and to perform basic life support functions as needed. If good scene and patient assessments are done, the EMT-Basic may know what the specific poison is and be in a better position to begin treatment while en route to the emergency room.

Poisoning and Scene Assessment

The EMT-Basic should be proactive in trying to determine why the patient is presenting with specific symptoms, as this investigation may well be the difference between a successful outcome and sudden patient death. For example, if you arrive at the scene of woman down, and the patient is unconscious in her bed with bradypnea, bradycardia, pale and diaphoretic and unresponsive, she could be the victim of a number of medical problems. If the EMT-Basic notices an empty pill bottle of Seconal™ next to the bed, he or she may then suspect a barbiturate overdose and notify the receiving facility of this finding, which will expedite treatment in the ER. Without this crucial piece of evidence, the receiving facility will have to perform a wide range of tests, and the critical element of time crucial to the patient's survival may be lost.

Treatment of Poisonings

Treatment of suspected poisonings will follow the usual protocol of assessing and treating the basic life-support functions. If the poison is known, basic protocols may allow treatments in the prehospital setting with proper medical control. Some jurisdictions, for example, allow the use by EMT-Basics of an emetic such as ipecac, a drug that will induce vomiting. This may be indicated for a patient who is known to have ingested a solid poison, such as sleeping pills, and if symptoms have not yet occurred. If the pills can be vomited out of the patient, then absorption into the patient's bloodstream will be prevented. Because of the dangers associated with managing the airway of a patient who is actively vomiting, many physicians are hesitant to allow the use of emetics by EMT-Basics, and would rather perform a gastric lavage in the emergency room, which involves insertion of a orogastric or nasogastric tube, irrigation of the stomach with saline, withdrawal of the stomach contents by suctioning the tube, and administration of activated charcoal to absorb any remaining toxins.

Oral administration of activated charcoal may also be indicated by a physician to an EMT-Basic, depending on the poison and the amount of time since ingestion. Activated charcoal is ground charcoal in a suspension of water forming aqueous slurry. Care in administration of activated charcoal should be exercised, since its ingestion, in spite of its relatively benign effects, may cause vomiting that is contraindicated.

Vomiting is not indicated if the poison is caustic, corrosive, or a petroleum product. These poisons will cause more damage to the esophageal passage as they come back up, and as such are better treated by being neutralized in the stomach. Petroleum products may also cause problems in the lungs if their vapors are aspirated.

Emergency care for poisoning and overdose involves good basic life support: maintaining an airway, adequate oxygen perfusion, and circulatory support, if necessary. A complete initial assessment followed by a comprehensive focused assessment is crucial to good prehospital care. As always, scene safety is crucial. For example, in the case of bee sting, if the bees are still swarming, then the scene is not safe and should not be entered unless the EMT-Basic is wearing suitable protective equipment. If the EMT-Basic is safe, then the patient must be removed as expeditiously as possible from the unsafe condition. Carbon-monoxide poisoning is another such case. The EMT-Basic must be aware of the lethality of the odorless gas in a closed space. If the scene is safe, the EMT-Basic can transport the poisoned individual to a receiving facility with a hyperbaric chamber, a device helpful in carbon-monoxide poisoning.

Another aspect of a complete assessment is to bring the receiving facility any identifying containers or labels. These may contain the chemical information necessary for treatment, as well as indicate the amount of the poison taken in by the patient.

ENVIRONMENTAL EMERGENCIES

The human body consistently maintains an internal temperature of approximately 98.6 degrees Fahrenheit in order to function properly. If the body gives off more heat than it generates, this leads to a condition referred to as hypothermia, or low body temperature. The body may lose heat by five different mechanisms: radiation, convection, conduction, evaporation, and breathing.

Hypothermia

Hypothermia, or heat loss, is a common situation. The EMT-Basic must be familiar with its mechanisms, signs, and symptoms, and care.

Mechanisms of Heat Loss Causing Hypothermia

The following mechanisms cause heat loss:

- Radiation is when heat is given off into an area or object that has a lower temperature than the radiating object. A person standing outdoors in subfreezing temperatures radiates heat to the surrounding cold atmosphere, primarily through the extremities.

- Convection is the process by which heat is given off into adjacent cold molecules. As these are heated, they are replaced with cold molecules. An example of convection is wind chill. Studies have shown that exposed flesh will freeze in less than a minute at minus 70 degrees Fahrenheit. While this situation does not occur normally in the continental United States, a temperature of minus 20 degrees Fahrenheit with a wind of 25 to 30 mph will be the equivalent of minus 70 degrees, which is a fairly normal winter condition in the northern United States.

- Conduction is when heat is passed through a colder object by direct contact. Water will conduct heat 240 times faster than air, which is why a subject immersed in cold water is subject to rapid hypothermia.

- Evaporation is when liquid is heated to a gaseous state, causing a loss of temperature. This is the process of perspiring, which is one of the regulatory mechanisms a body uses to maintain normal temperature.

- The respiratory process, in which air heated by the body is exhaled into the atmosphere and replaced with cooler ambient air, also causes a loss of temperature.

Signs and Symptoms of Hypothermia

As stated earlier, hypothermia is caused by a loss of body temperature, such as being in a cold environment without suitable clothing, for example, or by rapid immersion in cold water. Gradual hypothermia progresses through five stages:

- In the first stage, the body shivers as it attempts to raise its core temperature by the activity.

- In the second stage, there is mental apathy and loss of motor functions.

- In the third stage there is a decreased level of responsiveness and freezing of the extremities.

- In the fourth stage, the vital signs begin to decrease and slow.

- Finally, in the fifth stage of hypothermia, death occurs.

In assessing for hypothermia, the EMT-Basic should feel the patient's torso or abdomen, which will be the best indicator for a low core body temperature. If it feels cold to the touch, then the examiner must check and note if verbal responses and motor responses are normal or if they are impaired, and if so, to what degree. If shivering is present, then the patient may be in stage-one hypothermia; if absent, the patient may have already passed through stage one and entered into stage two or three. As hypothermia progresses, skin color will initially be red and then will become pale and finally cyanotic. It will also become stiff and hard in the latter stages. Note that the extremely young and the extremely old are especially susceptible to hypothermia.

Emergency Care for Hypothermia

Care for the patient, with hypothermia begins with his or her removal from the cold environment and removal of any wet clothing. Supplemental oxygen should be given at the highest level tolerated by the patient, and the patient should be gradually warmed by the use of blankets and warm water bottles to the groin, axillary, and cervical regions. The ambient temperature of the truck should be raised as the patient is transported.

Localized cold injuries, or frostbite, will begin in the extremities and in any areas with poor circulation. The skin will initially turn white and progress to a waxy look as the injury progresses. It will feel frozen and rigid upon palpation, and swelling and blisters may be present. To minimize damage, splinting of the extremity may be considered, and the extremity should be gradually rewarmed. If there is a long or delayed transport, the EMT-Basic should consider rewarming the extremity with a warm water bath. The EMT-Basic must be aware that the patient will complain of severe pain as the injured extremity begins to thaw.

Hyperthermia

The opposite of hypothermia is overheating, or hyperthermia, in which heat gained exceeds heat lost. This may lead to a potentially fatal increase in the core body temperature. There are three specific types of hyperthermia that the EMT-Basic must be aware of: heat cramps, heat exhaustion, and heatstroke.

- Heat cramps are muscle cramps caused by excessive body heat, and are not always due to strenuous activity. Cramps are usually the first indicator of hyperthermia and are often remedied by cooling the patient gradually.

- Heat exhaustion is characterized by general weakness and is accompanied by warm skin and profuse sweating. The patient should be removed to a cooler environment and placed in a semi-Fowler position for transport to a medical facility. The patient should be gradually cooled by increasing air-conditioning.

- Heatstroke is severe hyperthermia caused by a failure of the body's cooling mechanism. Heatstroke is marked by severely hot and dry skin and is a major medical emergency. The body's core temperature must be decreased immediately. In addition to basic life support, treatment should include aggressive cooling, including the use of cool wet towels to the groin, axillary, and cervical regions. These measures should be taken en route to the emergency room and should not delay transport.

Water Emergencies

Water emergencies present their own unique set of challenges to the EMT-Basic. Scene safety is always paramount, and no rescue should ever be attempted that is beyond the skill of the EMT-Basic. The decision to swim out to a subject who is drowning should only be undertaken by a suitably trained rescuer as a last resort. If an object can be extended to the victim or a flotation device thrown, or if there is a boat available, these should all be considered before anyone enters the water.

As with all situations in which the mechanism of injury is unknown, assume that the victim has suffered a traumatic injury and take the suitable spinal precautions. If the victim is breathing and has a pulse, consider placing him or her on a spine-board while he or she is still in the water.

A subject who has been immersed in cold water who presents with no breathing or pulse should be given CPR immediately, as the mammalian diving reflex may have placed the patient in a state of stasis. This reflex may have enabled the patient to have survived below the surface of the water. The state of Alaska currently recommends CPR if the patient has been in the water for less than one hour.

If there is a problem ventilating a patient due to abdominal distention, then the patient should be placed left lateral recumbent and gentle pressure applied to the abdomen to relieve the distention. Suction should be ready to assist in clearing the airway if fluid is vomited by this maneuver.

Bites and Stings

Bites and stings are treated as both wounds and possible injection poisonings. In addition, there is always the possibility of an allergic reaction. If the stinger is still present in the wound, it should be removed with tweezers or forceps and saved for the emergency room.

BEHAVIORAL EMERGENCIES

EMS is the default agency when emergencies do not fit into the departments of police or fire. In the early days of EMS, there was very little training in dealing with behavioral emergencies, yet EMS became the lead agency when the police, fire department, or civilians were confronted with a situation involving mental illness. Therefore, many EMS treatment regimens and protocols developed in response to these incidents after the fact. The National Standard Curriculum mandates that the EMT-Basic be able to define "behavior" and "behavioral emergency."

Defining Behavioral Emergencies

Behavior is defined in the curriculum as the "manner in which a person acts or performs; any or all activities of a person, including physical and mental activity." A behavioral emergency is defined as "a situation in which the patient exhibits abnormal behavior within a given situation that is unacceptable or intolerable to the patient, family, or community. This behavior can be due to extremes of emotion leading to violence or other inappropriate behavior, or due to a psychological or physical condition such as lack of oxygen or low blood sugar in diabetes.

The key words in the definition of behavioral emergency are "unacceptable" or "intolerable." This is oftentimes a subjective measurement. For example, walking down the street naked and singing a song may be perfectly acceptable in a nudist camp, but will likely lead to arrest and/or an EMS intervention in any city. The EMT-Basic must therefore be aware of the standards of behavior in the community in which he or she practices.

Some behaviors are obviously unacceptable or intolerable. Threatening to commit suicide or threatening to violently assault another person are clear examples of unacceptable behaviors. These may be conscious rational decisions, or they may be brought on in a normally healthy individual by a variety of physical conditions, including low blood sugar, anoxia, inadequate blood perfusion to the brain, head trauma, mind-altering substances, psychosis, excessive heat, and excessive cold. Furthermore, sometimes a perfectly rational and lucid patient with a common medical condition may suddenly become irrational and violent.

The good news is that most behavioral emergency calls are usually nonviolent. A patient may have a panic attack, in which he or she suddenly has an irrational fear of something, or the patient may simply be crying and unable to stop. But a mentally ill patient may quickly become violent, and the EMT-Basic must be prepared to react quickly to assure the safety of the EMS crew and the proper care and treatment of the patient.

Common Psychological Crises

Some of the common psychological crises that EMS may encounter include: anxiety or panic disorder, in which the patient becomes agitated or unreasonably fearful of current or future events; phobias, which are irrational fears of specific things, places, or situations; depression, or deep feelings of sadness, worthlessness, and discouragement with no sign of any relief; bipolar disorder, in which the patient alternates between moods of extreme euphoria and extreme depression (these stages may last a few minutes to months at a time); paranoia, in which the patient is fearful and mistrustful of everyone and everything; and schizophrenia, in which the patient can exhibit a wide variety of different symptoms, including delusions, thought disorders, blunted affect, or catatonia.

Any of these crises may present a danger to the patient, with an increased risk of bodily harm due to his or her engaging in risky or suicidal behaviors, or present a danger to bystanders and responding EMTs. As part of securing the scene and patient assessment, the EMT-Basic must be aware that a patient who paces nervously, shouts, threatens others, curses, throws objects, or stands grimacing with clenched fists has a greatly increased potential to suddenly turn violent. A patient who exhibits any of these signs or symptoms should be presumed to be capable of a sudden violent attack, and the EMT-Basic should be prepared to respond accordingly. Police support should be available for any call in which the EMT-Basic suspects there may be a behavioral problem.

Suicidal Behavior

The EMT-Basic should know which patients are at risk for suicidal behavior. It is common for patients who are in the throes of severe depression to decline medical intervention, which is their right unless they are impaired. Accordingly, a patient who is at an increased risk for suicide is presumed to not have the capacity to refuse medical treatment. If a patient says the words "I want to kill myself," it is important that the EMT-Basic not allow the patient to refuse transport to the local medical facility for an evaluation. However, often the patient will skate around the issue, so the EMT-Basic must decide whether the patient is actually at risk for a suicide attempt.

The following are indicators of an increased risk of suicide and must be taken seriously by the EMT-Basic in making the determination that a patient cannot refuse transportation. The risk factors include individuals over 40 who are single, widowed, or divorced, with a history of alcohol abuse and depression; patients who have a defined lethal plan of action that they will verbalize; an unusual gathering of articles that can cause death, i.e., guns, pills, ropes, etc.; a previous history of suicide attempts or behaviors; a recent diagnosis of serious illness; the recent loss of a significant loved one; and arrest, imprisonment, or loss of job.

As the EMT-Basic assesses a patient with any of these risk factors, it is important that he or she present a calm, and yet authoritative demeanor. The EMT-Basic should maintain eye contact and speak to the patient in a measured, calm tone. If the patient questions the EMT-Basic, the answers should be honest yet noninflammatory. It is better to attempt to defuse this pattern of thinking by not agreeing with everything the patient says, but by pointing out options and positive things, such as the concern of the patient's family. If the patient is delusional or hallucinating, assure the patient that the symptoms are not real.

Restraints

Behavioral calls are normally longer in duration than others, as the EMT-Basic often has to get the patient to cooperate in transportation to the medical facility. Yet in spite of all of the EMT-Basic's best efforts, it is sometimes necessary to forcefully restrain a patient.

Local protocols vary in the use of restraints. Some jurisdictions limit the application of restraints to police, some allow EMS to restrain patients with medical control approval, and others allow EMS to restrain if it can document a clear threat. Local protocols should always be followed, since the alternative may be a charge against the EMT-Basic for assault, battery, and/or false imprisonment.

If EMS is authorized to restrain a violent patient, then a minimum of five people are necessary for the safe application of leather, cloth, or vinyl restraints, one for each limb and one to apply the restraints. A patient should never be restrained in a prone position with ankles drawn up, the so-called "hog-tie." Many deaths due to asphyxia have been documented of patients in this type of restraint.

Police often deliver patients to EMS with their wrists secured behind their backs with handcuffs and their ankles in leg irons secured to the handcuffs. Police will routinely subdue violent patients with this technique in a prone position. If this patient is then delivered into EMS care, the EMT-Basic must immediately place the patient on his or her side in a lateral recumbent position to preclude asphyxia. The use of metal restraints (handcuffs and leg irons) is discouraged by current EMS standards due to the danger of violent patients causing damage to their tendons and ligaments as they struggle against the restraints. These restraints, however, with their ease of use and application, are often much safer to apply than leather and vinyl ones. A patient in metal restraints should be shifted to softer restraints once a sufficient number of personnel are available to safely accomplish this change.

Restraint Procedures

With a person on each limb, the patient is then forced to a supine position on a backboard. Restraint cuffs are placed on each ankle and then secured to the backboard to prevent kicking. A strap is used to secure the patient's legs just above the knees, then another strap across the chest just below the armpits. A restraint cuff is applied to each wrist, and the arms crossed over the chest and restrained to the backboard.

An alternative to this method is to restrain the wrists with the nondominant hand (if known) tractioned along the side of the body and the dominant hand secured to the top of the backboard above the patient's head. The advantages to this method are that the patient's torso is clear. If chest compressions suddenly have to be performed, the EMT-Basic can observe the patient's diaphragm for signs of respiratory distress, and the patient's arm is available for an IV if one becomes necessary. The disadvantage is that the patient is not as secure as he or she would be if the arms were crossed over the chest, helping to hold them in the supine position. Remember to constantly assess the patient's respiratory function as well as distal circulation, as these may quickly become impaired because of the restraints.

To reiterate, local medical protocols must always be followed. Behavioral emergencies, because of their medical and legal complexities, must be thoroughly documented, both as to observation of the patient and EMS interactions. Any medical-control permissions must be documented completely as to the individual giving permission for specific actions and the time of permission. Since complaints against EMTs are common in these situations, it is important that the names of witnesses, assisting EMTs, and police officers are also well documented.

OBSTETRIC AND GYNECOLOGICAL EMERGENCIES

Childbirth is a natural process, and the EMT-Basic's role is one of support, as well as being able to recognize abnormal situations and work to correct them. As with medical emergencies and trauma, the EMT-Basic must be aware of the special anatomy and physiology of the pregnant female and her unborn child.

Pregnancy and Childbirth

The unborn child is called a fetus and lives in the uterus, or womb, of the mother. Once a female's ovum (egg) is fertilized by a male sperm, it begins to grow and divide into multiple cells and implants itself in the wall of the uterus, where it will be nourished. The normal period for gestation is 36 weeks from the time of ovum fertilization. The opening of the uterus into the birth canal or vagina, is called the cervix. This opening is blocked by a mucus plug during pregnancy which is discharged as labor begins and the cervix begins to dilate in preparation of delivery of the fetus.

In addition to the fetus, the uterus also contains a developing organ called the placenta, which is the organ through which the fetus receives nourishment and to which the fetus is connected by the umbilical cord. A sac of amniotic fluid (bag of waters) surrounds the fetus while in utero to cushion and protect the fetus. This sac will usually rupture on its own; this is often the precursor of active labor. Occasionally the sac will deliver unruptured with the baby and must be torn by the EMT-Basic to enable the baby to breathe. Crowning is when the baby's head is visible in the birth canal.

The perineum is the area between a female's vagina and anus. This is commonly torn during the delivery of a fetus. In a hospital setting, an obstetrician or midwife may cut this area before crowning to expedite delivery. This procedure is called an episiotomy; the perineum is then stitched after birth to facilitate healing.

Labor

Labor is the process of delivery of a fetus and is defined as beginning with the first pronounced uterine contraction and terminating with the delivery of the placenta. It is subdivided into three stages:

- The first stage of labor occurs as contractions begin and may last from a few minutes to many hours. The contractions can be palpated on the mother's abdomen. These contractions cause the cervix to dilate in preparation for the baby's expulsion from the uterus.
- The second stage of labor is reached when the cervix is fully dilated and the baby's head begins to enter the birth canal. It is at this stage that the EMT-Basic should be able to observe the baby's head during the contraction. This stage culminates with the delivery of the baby.
- The third stage of labor is the delivery of the placenta.

The first part of the baby that is visible is referred to as the presenting part and usually will be the baby's head. If any other part of the baby presents first, this is referred to as a breech delivery.

Each EMS unit should carry an obstetrical kit, which should consist of surgical scissors, two hemostats or cord clamps, umbilical tape or sterilized cord bulb syringe, sterile towels, 2 × 10 gauze sponges, sterile gloves, one sterile baby blanket, sanitary napkins, and a biohazard plastic bag. These kits may be preassembled, or standard prepackaged kits may be purchased.

Obstetrical Assessment

Assessment of a patient in labor is the same as any other medical assessments with the following additions. It is useful to know which pregnancy this is for the mother. A first pregnancy will usually have a longer labor period than a fourth or fifth pregnancy. The patient or a bystander should also be asked if her prior pregnancies have ended in live births or miscarriages, whether the live births were vaginal deliveries or Caesarean sections, and whether there were any specific complications with her prior births. It is important to note that some women may deny that they are pregnant due to social stigma or other concerns, and the EMT-Basic may have to rely on his or her own observations as to whether an obstetrical emergency exists. If the patient is in active labor, the EMT-Basic must ask how far apart the contractions are and how long they last. The longer the contractions and the more frequently they occur, the more likely that delivery is imminent.

Miscarriage

The EMT-Basic must be aware of the predelivery emergency conditions that may be encountered. The first is spontaneous abortion or miscarriage. A miscarriage is when the products of conception are delivered early in the pregnancy. This will usually be dispatched as "woman bleeding or hemorrhaging." The assessment and care of the patient will be the same as for any patient with severe hemorrhaging. If the products of conception are available, they should be placed in a plastic bag and transported to the hospital out of the sight of the mother for the obstetrician to evaluate.

A miscarriage is an emotionally traumatic event for the family, and prehospital care for the emotional trauma is as important as the physical care. The EMT must be supportive and encouraging, just as he or she would be if a patient's loved one had died. The pain of loss should not be minimized by the EMT-Basic because the loss is not a fully developed human being. Statements like "You can always have another child" are minimizing statements and may not even be true. Support is often best given by conveying your concern and sense of loss to the mother.

Complications in Pregnancy

Seizures during pregnancy should always be treated as a major medical emergency. Once the patient has been properly assessed, she should be transported as expeditiously as possible. When transporting a pregnant woman, it is always preferable to transport her left lateral recumbent to allow for the best possible blood flow and to avoid constricting the inferior vena cava.

Vaginal bleeding during pregnancy is always considered serious, whether or not accompanied by abdominal pain. Bleeding can be controlled by application of sanitary napkins to the external vagina, and transport should be expedited.

A pregnant woman subjected to trauma is treated like any other trauma victim, with special attention paid to the abdomen and vagina for signs of bleeding. If immobilization is indicated, the patient is packaged in accordance with local protocols and the spine board is tilted to the left by placing pillows beneath the right side of the board. If spinal immobilization is not indicated, than the patient should be transported on her left side.

Emergency Procedures for Delivery

If the call is for a normal first-stage labor patient and delivery does not appear to be imminent based upon the primary assessment, then the EMT-Basic must complete the secondary assessment and determine if there is enough time to transport the patient safely to the hospital or if it would be safer to deliver the baby at the current location. This decision should be made in consultation with medical control, which will want to know specific symptoms and vital signs.

If the baby is crowning and delivery is imminent, the EMT-Basic should open the emergency obstetrics kit and prepare for delivery. Proper BSI precautions include sterile gloves, mask, gown, and eye protection. The procedures are as follows:

- The mother should lie on her back in a semi-Fowler position, propped up with pillows and with her knees drawn up and spread apart. Elevate the mother's buttocks with blankets or pillows.

- Create a sterile field around the vagina using paper barriers or towels. Do not touch the mother's vagina except during delivery if necessary to maintain the baby's airway, and even then only when your partner is present.

- As the baby's head is delivered, apply gentle pressure on the skull to prevent explosive delivery, avoiding the baby's fontanel, or soft spot.

- If the amniotic sac is still intact, puncture it and pull it away from the baby's mouth and nose as they appear.

- As the baby's head is delivered, check that the cord is not wrapped around the neck. If it is, try and unwrap it. If that it not possible, clamp the cord and cut it between the clamps.

- After the head is delivered, support the head with one hand and suction the mouth and nose two or three times with the bulb syringe. The torso and the rest of the body will usually be delivered with the next contraction. As the feet are delivered, grab the feet with one hand and wipe the blood and mucus from the mouth and nose with sterile gauze.

- If the baby is breathing normally, wrap the baby in a warm blanket, being sure to cover the baby's head to minimize heat loss. Place the baby on its side, the head slightly lower than the trunk. The baby should be level with the mother's vagina until the cord is cut.

- With the baby stable, and if the cord was not wrapped around the neck and cut already, clamp the cord three to four inches from the baby and cut the cord between the clamps once the pulsations of the cord have ceased.

- If the baby and the mother are stable, the EMT-Basic should prepare to deliver the placenta. As the uterus contracts, the EMT should urge the mother to push and expel the placenta. Once the placenta is delivered, place the placenta in the plastic bag and transport it along with the baby and mother to the hospital. The obstetrician will want to examine the placenta to be sure that all of it was expelled.

- Place two sanitary napkins over the vagina and have the mother close her legs. Have the mother massage her uterus through her abdomen to assist in the control of bleeding.

- If the mother begins to exhibit signs of shock (pale and diaphoretic), administer oxygen via nonrebreather and expedite transport.

APGAR Score

Patient assessment of a neonate (newborn baby) includes the APGAR score, which should be performed at one minute postpartum and five minutes postpartum. This index gives an excellent overall summary of the baby's condition and will alert the receiving hospital to the actual condition. APGAR stands for **A**ppearance, **P**ulse, **G**rimace, **A**ctivity, and **R**espirations. It is a good idea to have this scorecard posted on the action wall of the truck. The maximum score is 10 and the minimum score is 0, with 0 to 2 points assessed for each part.

- **A**ppearance: if the baby's extremities are pink, assign two points; if the torso is pink but the extremities bluish, assign one point; if the entire baby is cyanotic or pale, zero points.

- **P**ulse: if the heart rate is greater than 100, assign two points; if less than 100, assign one point; if no pulse, zero points.

- **G**rimace: if you flick the soles of the neonate's feet and the baby grimaces, coughs, sneezes, or cries, two points; if there is only some slight facial grimace, one point; if no response to your stimulation, zero points.

- **A**ctivity: If the baby is actively moving around, two points; if only some flexion of extremities, one point; if no movement and limp, zero points.

- **R**espirations: If the baby displays good respirations and a strong cry, two points; if slow and irregular breathing effort with a weak cry, one point; if no respirations, zero points.

The number of personnel available may dictate that this assessment not be done; for example, a finding of no respirations should lead the EMT-Basic to begin respiratory assistance and not to be recording assessment findings. An APGAR of 7 to 10 is considered good; an APGAR of 4 to 6 indicates a neonate that is moderately depressed, and stimulation and oxygen are indicated; an APGAR of 0 to 3 indicates aggressive resuscitation, including positive ventilation and chest compressions.

Abnormal Delivery

Abnormal delivery situations are rare, but still are a concern to the EMT-Basic. Some recommended EMT intervention situations include prolapsed cord, breech birth, meconium aspiration, and premature birth.

Prolapsed cord is a condition in which the cord presents from the vagina before the head of the baby is delivered. This presents a serious emergency for the viability of the fetus. Treatment for this condition, in addition to normal assessment and oxygenation for the mother, includes placing the mother's head below her buttocks to lessen pressure on the birth canal and fetus. If the cord is still pulsating, insert a gloved hand into the vagina and push the presenting part of the fetus away from the cord to prevent the pressure of the neonate from cutting off the flow of blood through the cord. Transport immediately and continue to monitor the pulsation of the cord.

As discussed earlier, a breech presentation is where any part of the fetus other than the head presents through the birth canal first. This requires immediate transport upon recognition. The mother should be placed on high-flow oxygen and transported in a head down position with her pelvis elevated.

Meconium aspiration occurs when a neonate, due to distress during labor, defecates into the amniotic fluid and then aspirates this fluid as it begins to breathe. The presence of meconium is detectable when the amniotic fluid is greenish or yellowish brown instead of clear. If meconium is detected, the EMT-Basic should aspirate the oropharynx before trying to stimulate spontaneous respirations.

Premature babies, before the full 36-week gestation period, are especially at risk for hypothermia, so these infants must be kept warm, especially the crowns of their head, so that they can retain heat. Early premature infants—less than 30 weeks—will also usually require manual resuscitation.

Gynecological Emergencies

Gynecological emergencies also present special considerations, especially for male EMT-Basics who may be sensitive or embarrassed by treating female genitalia. Severe vaginal bleeding is treated in the same way as any other internal hemorrhage, with oxygen and immediate transport.

Special sensitivity is required in dealing with women who have been sexually assaulted. It is always preferable to have a female EMT, if possible, be the primary caregiver as the victim may be fearful of any male at this time, especially those in uniform who are projecting an image of power. The primary EMT, whether male or female, must be nonjudgmental in dealing with the victim of sexual assault, which requires thorough professionalism as well as a supportive attitude.

In addition to following the normal trauma assessment protocols, it is important to preserve any evidence for possible criminal prosecution. The patient must be discouraged from showering, bathing, or voiding if at all possible. Visual examination of the genitalia should only be conducted if profuse bleeding is present. Some states require medical practitioners, including EMT-Basics, to report any sexual assault they become aware of.

PRACTICE SET

1. What medication is not indicated for the EMT-Basic treatment of chest pain?

   (A) Nitroglycerin

   (B) Aspirin

   (C) Oxygen

   (D) Epinephrine

2. Which of the following is not a drug?

   (A) Oxygen

   (B) Aspirin

   (C) Oral glucose

   (D) AED

3. Which of the following is one of the five "Rights" to be observed when administering drugs?

   (A) Right to remain silent

   (B) Right of refusal

   (C) Right date

   (D) Right of explanation

4. You respond to a call for difficulty breathing. Arriving on scene, you find a male in his sixties breathing rapidly and sitting in tripod position. His color is bluish, and he is sweaty and cool to the touch. You perform your initial assessment, which is unremarkable, and his vital signs are all within normal range except for his respiratory rate, which is 22. What is your first medication of choice to treat this patient?

   (A) Epinephrine

   (B) Albuterol

   (C) Nitroglycerin

   (D) Oxygen

5. In the scenario in question 4, what device, dosage, and route would you use to administer the drug?

   (A) .3 mg epinephrine via subcutaneous injection

   (B) 2 liters per minute oxygen via nasal cannula

   (C) 12 liters per minute oxygen via non-rebreather mask

   (D) 1 dose albuterol via metered inhaler

6. Which of the following signs and symptoms is indicative of inadequate air exchange?

   (A) Breath sounds clear in all fields

   (B) Chest rises and falls with each breath

   (C) Respiratory rate between 12 and 20 times per minute

   (D) Altered mental status

7. You arrive on the scene of a call for difficulty breathing. You enter the kitchen and you see a seventy-year-old male seated at the table leaning forward. He is having severe trouble breathing, his skin is bluish-gray, and he is sweaty. You hear a gurgling sound as he tries to inhale. As you ask him questions, he tries to respond between gasps, but his answers are not comprehensible. He is clutching his chest and appears to be in severe pain. His wife advises you that he had a heart attack last year and takes nitroglycerin, hydrochlorothiazide, and digitalis. The chest pains began as he finished supper. The patient took two NTG tablets, but the pain has continued to get worse. His vital signs are BP 180/120, pulse 120, respiratory rate 28, pulse oximetry 82 percent. What is your next intervention?

   (A) Load and go

   (B) Oxygen 15 lpm via nonrebreather

   (C) Contact medical control for NTG 1:150 sublingually

   (D) Apply the AED and analyze his cardiac rhythm

8. You have made the load-and-go decision on the patient in question 7 and remove him immediately to the truck after you've applied the oxygen mask at high flow. As you begin your focused exam en route to the hospital, you notice your patient is now unconscious and has stopped breathing, and you cannot palpate a carotid pulse. You instruct your partner to begin ventilating the patient with a BVM and OPA, and hook up the AED to the patient. You ask the driver to stop while you analyze the patient with the AED. The AED reads "no shock advised." Which of the following statements is correct as your next action?

(A) Bypass the automated feature on the AED and deliver 200 joules countershock.

(B) Contact medical control for permission to administer NTG 1:150 sublingually.

(C) Continue transport with no further intervention.

(D) Begin chest compressions for one minute and then reanalyze with the AED.

9. You are dispatched to a call for a man down. You arrive on scene and find a male in his seventies lying on his back on the front lawn. There are no bystanders or family members present. He is cyanotic, pulseless, and apneic. He is cool to the touch, and when you try to move his limbs and jaw, they are rigid and do not move. You pull his shirt up and notice that the anterior portion of his torso is pale and the posterior is black-and-blue, with a definitive line between the two areas. Which of the following conditions should you suspect?

(A) Cardiac arrest

(B) Myocardial infarction

(C) Apnea secondary to COPD

(D) Biological death

10. You are dispatched to a residence for a female with a possible heart attack. You respond priority and arrive on scene. The scene is safe, and you are wearing appropriate protective gear. You find a forty-four-year-old female sitting in the living room with her right hand on her upper chest. She is conscious, alert, and oriented times three, and appears to be in no apparent distress. She states that she has a dull pain in her midchest area that does not radiate and is approximately 4 on the 10 scale. Her color appears normal, and she is not diaphoretic. Which of the following is not an appropriate intervention?

(A) Oxygen

(B) Aspirin

(C) AED

(D) CPR

11. Which of the following medical terms is generally referred to as a "heart attack"?

(A) Amyotropic Lateral Sclerosis

(B) Cerebral vascular accident

(C) Myocardial infarction

(D) Menses interruptus

12. You are dispatched to the front lawn of a residence for a possible heart attack. You respond priority and arrive on scene wearing the proper protective equipment. The scene is safe, and you see a male in his mid-eighties lying supine on the lawn. He appears unresponsive and cyanotic with his mouth and eyes open. You perform an airway maneuver, and he has no spontaneous respirations; you cannot detect a carotid pulse. What is your next procedure?

(A) Ask bystanders to call 911.

(B) Request an ALS intercept.

(C) Perform CPR.

(D) Administer 325 mg aspirin PO.

13. Ventricular fibrillation is a condition affecting which system of the heart?

    (A) Electrical

    (B) Circulatory

    (C) Mechanical

    (D) All of the above

14. Which is the proper procedure for correction of the condition in question 13 by an EMT-Basic?

    (A) IV administration of lidocaine

    (B) Countershock by AED

    (C) Countershock by manual defibrillator at 200 joules

    (D) CPR

15. You are dispatched to a call for a man down. You arrive on scene and find a male in his seventies lying on his back on the front lawn. There are no bystanders or family members present. He is cyanotic, pulseless, and apneic. He is cool to the touch, and when you try to move his limbs and jaw they are rigid and do not move. You pull his shirt up and notice that the anterior portion of his torso is pale and the posterior is black-and-blue, with a definitive line between the two areas. Which of the following conditions should you suspect?

    (A) Cardiac arrest

    (B) Myocardial infarction

    (C) Apnea secondary to COPD

    (D) Biological death

16. You are dispatched to a college dorm room for a report of a man down. You respond priority and arrive on scene with suitable protective equipment and have determined that the scene is safe. You find an eighteen-year-old-male lying on his back, unconscious and not responsive to any stimuli. He has an airway and is making snoring sounds at a regular rate. As you are checking his breathing, you notice that his breath has a fruity odor. His carotid pulse is strong, rapid, and regular. His girlfriend is also in the room and is hysterical as she tells you they were sitting talking when he suddenly collapsed. What question do you want to ask the girlfriend next?

    (A) "Does he have any allergies?"

    (B) "Is he diabetic?"

    (C) "Is this a frequent occurrence?"

    (D) "Does he take any medications on a regular basis?"

17. In the scenario in question 16, the girlfriend answers that he is an insulin-dependent diabetic and takes insulin twice a day. He has just returned from competing in a triathlon, in which he regularly participates. Which drug do you want to consider next?

    (A) Oxygen

    (B) Oral glucose

    (C) Glucagon

    (D) Epinephrine

18. Which of the following conditions may cause a seizure?

    (A) High body temperature

    (B) Head injury

    (C) Epilepsy

    (D) All of the above

19. The most important procedure for an EMT-Basic to perform in dealing with a seizure patient is to

    (A) Secure the airway.
    (B) Secure the patient's limbs with restraints.
    (C) Administer 10 mg diazepam IM.
    (D) Transport priority.

20. You are dispatched to a restaurant for a report of difficulty breathing. You respond priority wearing appropriate protective equipment, and there are no scene safety concerns. You are directed to a table where a male and a female are seated. The female has her hand to her throat and appears to be in respiratory distress. She is moving air with difficulty, and her male companion is upset. She is unable to answer your questions, and her companion knows of no medical history, medications, or allergies. He advises that she had just eaten a shrimp cocktail when the symptoms suddenly developed. The patient is pale and diaphoretic, with a rapid pulse. The police officer who searched her pocketbook for her driver's license hands you an EpiPen™ that he found in the pocketbook. What should you do at this point?

    (A) Call medical control.
    (B) Administer the EpiPen™.
    (C) Administer oxygen via nonrebreather mask at 15 liters per minute.
    (D) Place the patient on a stretcher and transport priority to the nearest medical facility.

21. You are on duty in your station when a male subject comes running in. He is pale, diaphoretic, and short of breath. He keeps stammering the word "bee" and is pointing to his arm, where you notice a large welt. He is unable to respond to your questions and is beginning to lose consciousness. What condition do you suspect?

    (A) Anaphylaxis
    (B) Diabetes
    (C) Myocardial infarction
    (D) Epilepsy

22. You are dispatched to a residence for a possible overdose. You arrive on the scene and find police have secured the scene. You are wearing appropriate protective apparel. The husband advises that his wife has been despondent and he fears she may have overdosed on her prescription tranquilizers. He states that she has been drinking all day and is now semiconscious. In the bedroom you find a female in her fifties who appears to be sleeping. She is supine, making snoring sounds, and has a slow pulse. She responds when you call her name, but will not answer any questions. Her gaze is unfocused, and her pupils are dilated and do not respond to light. There is an empty bottle of Clonazepam™ next to the bed that was refilled yesterday and contained 30 one mg tablets. There is also an empty fifth of gin, and her breath smells of alcohol. Her husband states that she entered the bedroom 15 minutes before he called 911. Her vital signs are 100/60, respirations 12, and pulse 55. What is your next course of action?

    (A) Transport.
    (B) Contact medical control.
    (C) Administer 30 ml of syrup of ipecac followed by 16oz of water.
    (D) Administer 1,250 mg of activated charcoal.

23. You are dispatched to meet the police at a residence with no other information available. You arrive on scene and police lead you to a subject seated in his car, which is parked in his garage. The officer tells you that when they arrived the garage door was closed and the car was running. Police have shut the engine off and left the doors open. You enter the garage and observe a male seated behind the wheel of a car. He is unconscious and not responding to any stimuli. He is cyanotic, with slow, shallow respirations and a weak, thready pulse. What should you suspect as the cause of his unconsciousness?

    (A) Heart attack
    (B) Seizure
    (C) Cerebral thrombosis
    (D) Carbon-monoxide poisoning

24. In the scenario in question 23, as you arrive and meet with the police officer, what determination should you have initially made with the information he has given you?

    (A) This is a load and go.

    (B) This is a crime scene that must be preserved.

    (C) The scene is unsafe.

    (D) This call needs an Advanced Life Support unit.

25. In the scenario in question 23, you find the victim has been extricated to the front lawn by firefighters prior to EMS arrival. You have performed your assessments, and the vital signs are blood pressure 110/80, pulse 50, respirations 12 and shallow, and pulse oximeter shows that his oxygen saturation is 98 percent. What should be your next intervention?

    (A) Administer 30 ml of syrup of ipecac.

    (B) Administer 15 lpm oxygen.

    (C) Administer 4 mg morphine sulfate IM.

    (D) Administer .3 mg epinephrine by EpiPen™.

26. In the scenario in question 25, which piece of specialized equipment might influence your choice of destination hospital?

    (A) Heart-lung machine

    (B) Hyperbaric chamber

    (C) Antimatter drive

    (D) Positive pressure ventilator

27. Which of the following poisons should not be vomited?

    (A) Sulfuric acid

    (B) Lye

    (C) Kerosene

    (D) All of the above

28. You arrive on the scene of a motor vehicle accident on a cold snowy evening. The outside temperature is zero degrees Fahrenheit. You observe a subject lying in the snow next to a wrecked car. Police are on scene and you are wearing appropriate protective gear. The patient is a thirty-five-year-old male, semiconscious, breathing rapidly and with a weak thready pulse. You detect the odor of alcohol on his breath. As you palpate his torso, beneath his shirt you notice he is cold to the touch, but is not shivering. His hands and feet feel cold and rigid. Which stage of hypothermia do you suspect?

    (A) First stage

    (B) Second stage

    (C) Third stage

    (D) Fourth stage

29. In the scenario in question 28, you find two additional patients who have been ejected from the car and who present the same symptoms. One is a seventy-eight-year-old female and the other is a thiry-two-year-old female. Which of the following should be treated first?

    (A) thirty-five-year-old male

    (B) seventy-eight-year-old female

    (C) thirty-two-year-old female

    (D) Treatment should occur at the receiving facility.

30. In the scenario in question 29, you have removed the seventy-eight-year-old female to your truck and have begun transport. In addition to her lethargy, her vital signs are beginning to drop. You notice that her right hand was not gloved and now appears whitish and waxy. Which of the following treatments would be appropriate for this patient?

    (A) Warm packs under her arms, beneath her neck, and between her legs

    (B) Warm water bath for her right hand

    (C) Oxygen

    (D) All of the above

31. You are standing by a summer road race and are summoned to a runner who has fallen. The patient is an eighteen-year-old female who is lying underneath a tree, clutching her right leg. She is breathing rapidly and is flushed. Her skin is hot and dry. Which of the following conditions do you suspect and should you treat first?

    (A) Heat cramps

    (B) Heat exhaustion

    (C) Heatstroke

    (D) Heat conduction

32. You are en route back to quarters from the hospital when you observe a subject in the water 100 feet from a lake shore and appearing to be in distress. You notify your dispatcher and stand on the shore. The subject is flailing his arms and yelling, "Help!" Your own swimming ability is limited, and your partner cannot swim at all. What should be your next course of action?

    (A) Strip to your underwear and dive in, swimming to the victim as quickly as possible.

    (B) Wade into the water and attempt to throw him the rescue rope from the truck.

    (C) Drive back to quarters and get a boat.

    (D) Buddy-swim with your partner to the victim.

33. You are dispatched to a residence for an unknown-type medical call. You arrive on scene and determine that the scene is safe. You are wearing appropriate precautions. An adult female tells you she was working in her garden when she felt a stinging sensation on the back of her left arm. She is conscious, alert, and oriented times three with normal respirations and pulse. She has no significant medical history and no known allergies. You examine her left arm and see a bright red area five inches in diameter with a white spot in the center and a small black speck in the center of the white spot. What is your next course of action?

    (A) Contact medical control.

    (B) Administer epinephrine 1/1000.3 mg SQ.

    (C) Remove the black speck with tweezers.

    (D) Administer oxygen 10 liters per minute via nonrebreather mask.

34. You are dispatched to a residence for a woman in labor. You arrive on scene, having taken the usual precautions, and observe a female in her early thirties lying on the couch in the living room. She advises you that this is her third pregnancy, her bag of waters ruptured 30 minutes ago, and her pains are increasing in intensity and are currently three minutes apart. Which of the following should be your next move?

    (A) Place her on the stretcher and respond priority to the nearest maternity unit.

    (B) Tie her legs together to prevent premature birth and expedite transport.

    (C) Remove her underwear and, at the next contraction, examine the birth canal for signs of crowning.

    (D) Insert your hand into the birth canal and see if you can feel the baby's head.

35. In the scenario in question 34, you take vital signs and prepare for transport. The mother suddenly tells you she is having a contraction, and you observe the top of the baby's head as her labia separate. What should you now do?

    (A) Place her on the stretcher and respond priority to the nearest maternity unit.

    (B) Open the obstetrical kit and prepare for delivery.

    (C) Administer 15 lpm oxygen to the mother.

    (D) Allow nature to take its course.

36. In the scenario in question 34, instead of the top of the baby's head, you see the baby's arm protruding from the mother's vagina. What should you now prepare to do?

    (A) Place her on the stretcher and respond priority to the nearest maternity unit.

    (B) Open the obstetrical kit and prepare for delivery.

    (C) Pull gently on the arm to facilitate delivery.

    (D) Wait for the next contraction and see if the condition rectifies itself.

37. You are dispatched along with police to an unknown-type medical call. You arrive simultaneously with the police and observe a large male trying to throw a refrigerator at his wife. You assist police in wrestling the man to a prone position, and the police handcuff his wrists behind his back as he continues to struggle and curse. His wife advises you that he has no medical problems, takes no medication, and has no history of any psychological problems. She indicates he was behaving normally until she asked if he would like a cup of tea, at which point he suddenly assaulted her and became violent. The police place him under arrest and try to place him in a squad car. What is your role as the medical provider?

    (A) Assist the police in subduing and arresting the subject.

    (B) Intervene and demand that he be transported via rescue to the hospital.

    (C) Go back in service as this is a police matter.

    (D) Remove his restraints; place him on your stretcher and transport.

38. In the scenario in question 37, how should this patient be restrained by EMS?

    (A) Leave him in handcuffs and use leg irons to secure his ankles to his wrists in a prone position.

    (B) Place him in a supine position on a backboard and secure his limbs with leather or vinyl cuffs.

    (C) Place him a supine position on a backboard with his hands cuffed behind his back, place another backboard on top of him, and secure the backboards together with handcuffs.

    (D) Remove his metal restraints, wrap him in a blanket, and secure him to the stretcher with the stretcher straps.

39. You are dispatched to a college dorm for a possible diabetic emergency. You respond priority and arrive on scene. As you walk down the hallway, you observe a female whom you have previously treated for hypoglycemia secondary to diabetes talking and humming to herself. She is walking near the edge of a high balcony. Her roommates tell you that she has been behaving strangely all morning. What should be your next move?

    (A) Tackle her and restrain her.

    (B) Administer 1 mg glucagon IM.

    (C) Request police assistance.

    (D) Take her by the arm and gently sit her in a chair for a more thorough evaluation.

40. In the scenario in question 39, your evaluation reveals that the patient's answers are incoherent and inappropriate, her blood pressure is 120/80, her pulse is 72, and her respirations are 12. Her blood glucose is 76. She does not refuse to be transported and allows you to lead her to the truck where you place her in a semi-Fowler position and secure her to the stretcher with the normal straps. She now tries to unfasten the straps and pushes your arm away. What should you do?

    (A) Restrain her arms with soft restraints.

    (B) Handcuff her hands to the middle strap.

    (C) Place her on a backboard and secure her ankles to the board and her wrists above and to the side.

    (D) Contact medical control for permission to restrain.

ANSWER EXPLANATIONS

1. D

Epinephrine is indicated for treatment of anaphylaxis. All the other medications are used to treat chest pain.

2. D

The correct answer is (D) because oxygen, asprin, and glucose are all drugs. A drug is defined as any substance taken into the body to treat or prevent a disease or condition. The AED is a devce used to countershock a dysrhythmia and as such does not meet the definition.

3. C

It is the responsibility of the EMT-Basic acting under the specific protocol to assure that the medication being given has not passed its expiration date. The right to remain silent is a legal right against self-incrimination, and the right of refusal is a patient's legal right to refuse any medical procedure (including drug therapy), but is not one of the five rights listed for drug administration. Providing explanations is common practice, but is not an explicit right.

4. D

This patient is presenting signs of hypoxia and almost all state protocols allow the EMT-Basic to administer oxygen for immediate relief. Epinephrine is indicated for an allergic reaction, albuterol for airway obstruction, and nitroglycerin for chest pain. Be aware that albuterol may be indicated if the dyspnea is being caused by constricted bronchioles, but permission must first be obtained from medical control following a detailed assessment. Oxygen is always the first drug of choice in these situations.

5. C

The patient's condition requires high-flow oxygen (10–15 liters per minute), and the correct device to deliver this flow is the nonrebreather mask. Epinephrine is indicated for anaphylaxis, low-flow oxygen (2 lpm) would be indicated for mild hypoxia or dyspnea, and a metered inhaler for difficulty breathing caused by airway obstruction.

6. D

(D) is correct. (A), (B), and (C) are all indicative of normal respiratory pattern. Altered mental status may be caused by insufficient oxygen supply to the brain.

7. B

This patient is having severe difficulty breathing, and his pulse oximetry and skin color indicate hypoxia. This is a moderately difficult question, as all of the other answers could also be considered correct actions over the course of time. However, the question asks what your next course of action is, and this would be to try and relieve the hypoxia with supplemental oxygen therapy.

8. D

The current protocols require three no-shock advisories interspersed with one minute of CPR. EMT-Basics cannot bypass the automated feature of the AED without specific training and medical control. (B) is incorrect because the patient's problem at this time has progressed from chest pain to cardiac arrest. (C) also is incorrect, as protocols require CPR for this patient until ordered to discontinue by a physician.

9. D

This patient exhibits the signs and symptoms of rigor mortis and postmortem lividity, which will allow you in most jurisdictions to not perform CPR and turn this case over to law enforcement for investigation of sudden death. The cause of the sudden death may have been any of the other answers.

10. D

The patient obviously has a pulse and is breathing, as evidenced by her correct answers to the questions, and is conscious, alert, and oriented. (A), (B), and (C) are all appropriate treatments for chest pain, including the AED; you can explain to the patient that the latter is a precaution that will enable you to monitor her heart more closely.

11. C

The correct answer is myocardial infarction. Answer choice (A) is more commonly known as Lou Gehrig's disease, a progressive illness of the neuromuscular system. Answer choice (B) is a stroke. Answer choice (D) is a gynecological event.

12. C

The correct action is to perform CPR. Answer choice (A) is incorrect, since somebody has already called 911 and you are on scene. You should have requested the ALS intercept when dispatched to the possible heart call. Aspirin is indicated for chest pain, but this patient is unconscious and unresponsive and should not be given anything by mouth.

13. D

Ventricular fibrillation occurs when the electrical system of the heart no longer energizes the heart to pump properly and instead just vibrates (fibrillates) the cardiac muscle.

14. B

Countershock by AED is the correct answer. Answer choices (A) and (C) are Advanced Life Support procedures and (D), CPR, is indicated, but only if there is a delay in providing the AED countershock.

15. D

This patient exhibits the signs and symptoms of biological death, rigor mortis, and postmortem lividity, which will allow you in most jurisdictions to not perform CPR and turn this case over to law enforcement for investigation of sudden death. The cause of the sudden death may have been any of the other answers.

16. B

You should be considering diabetes because of the fruity odor of this patient's breath, which could be indicative of hypoglycemia. The key word in the question is "next." It is always important to fully read each question and each answer and find the one that is *most* appropriate.

17. C

Glucagon is the best answer. Oxygen and epinephrine are not indicated. Oral glucose is indicated under some systems, however, giving anything orally to an unconscious patient may induce vomiting and aspiration into the lungs. Glucagon intramuscular is the best choice in this scenario. Some systems also allow the use of portable glucometers to measure blood sugar level, which enables the EMT-Basic to make a more definitive diagnosis and treatment plan.

18. D

Any of the answers may cause a seizure.

19. A

Again, reading the question is very important. If you are answering a question on the NREMT examination dealing with medical emergencies, you can forget the basics. The question is what is the most important procedure, and the EMT-Basic must always be concerned with maintaining a patent airway. Securing the patient's limbs (B) may be a secondary consideration to provide for patient and crew safety and a priority transport (D) is probably indicated, but not the most important. (C) is an advanced life support treatment for continuing seizures, and the question specifically states "EMT-Basic." The EMT-Basic should be familiar with Advanced Life Support medications, however, and diazepam is the generic name for the more commonly known drug Valium™.

20. A

The EMT-Basic must contact medical control. Some jurisdictions do permit EpiPen™ use by basic EMTs without medical control, but most locations require permission. Supplemental oxygen will help the hypoxia, but, if the airway swells shut, then supplemental oxygen is useless. Also, quick transport may not be sufficient if the airway is closing quickly. This patient is suffering an acute allergic reaction to shellfish and needs epinephrine immediately.

21. A

The patient is probably having an allergic (anaphylactic) reaction to a bee sting, as evidenced by his symptoms and his repeating the word "bee." A diabetic emergency would cause him to lose consciousness, a myocardial infarction (heart attack) is usually accompanied by chest pains, and epilepsy is a condition that causes seizures followed by loss of consciousness.

22. A

This patient should be transported immediately. Answer choice (B) should be done while en route, and (C) and (D) may be appropriate after consultation with medical control.

23. D

Circumstances would indicate that a running car in a closed garage emitting carbon monoxide, a poison, has caused this condition, although the others cannot be ruled out initially.

24. C

EMS personnel should not enter this environment without proper respiratory protection, such as a self-contained breathing apparatus. To do so invites possible carbon-monoxide poisoning, which delays proper care to the initial patient and complicates the entire rescue by adding to the total number of victims who must be treated. Answer choices (A) and (B) might be correct if the scene were safe. Regarding (D), there is nothing in this scenario that would indicate the intervention of an ALS unit.

25. B

This patient is severely hypoxic as indicated by his physical appearance and high-flow oxygen therapy is indicated. The high pulse oximeter is grossly misleading in carbon-monoxide poisoning, as it gives a false high reading due to the presence of carbon monoxide in the red blood cells, and thus cannot be relied on in this case. If you didn't know that, you could still use process of elimination. Ipecac would be indicated for poison ingestion, not inhalation, morphine for pain management in the ALS setting only, and epinephrine for an allergic reaction.

26. B

The hyperbaric chamber, in which outside oxygen pressure is increased, has proven to be effective in treatment of carbon-monoxide poisoning. This decision may be made by protocol or medical control, but if the EMT-Basic is given the choice between two hospital emergency rooms, in this scenario he or she should go with the hospital with the hyperbaric chamber. Answer choice (A) is normal equipment for any hospital with a full operating suite and would not be necessary for treating carbon-monoxide poisoning. Answer choice (D) is standard equipment in any hospital emergency room, and answer choice (C) is the device in *Star Trek®* that enables warp speed.

27. D

Answer choices (A) and (B) are corrosives that should not be vomited, and answer choice (C) is a petroleum product and its vapors may be aspirated.

28. C

The absence of shivering means the patient has moved beyond stage one. Stage two is marked by increasing mental apathy and loss of motor function, but stage three is when the extremities begin to freeze. Stage four would be when his vital signs begin to drop, so the most correct answer is (C).

29. B

The elderly person is more at risk for increasing hypothermia due to her age.

30. D

The patient is in fourth-stage hypothermia and needs to be warmed. In addition, she has symptoms of frostbite to her right hand that can be treated en route with a warm water bath. Oxygen is indicated for this patient due to her increasing lethargy.

31. C

While answer choices (A) and (B) may seem correct, in reading the question you must be able to identify that heatstroke is the most serious of the three and the condition you should be concerned about. This patient has a high core temperature, and her body's heat-regulating mechanisms are not working, so she must be cooled down with cold packs to the axillary, cervical, and groin areas.

32. B

Never undertake a rescue unless you are confident in your abilities to perform the necessary activity. Since neither you nor your partner is trained in water rescue techniques, you should not attempt to swim to the patient. If you have an object to throw to the victim, this is your best course of action. Leaving the scene to go and get a boat could be considered abandonment of the patient, and since your partner cannot swim, a buddy swim is not a possibility, nor does it solve the problem of being able to approach and assist the victim.

33. C

The patient's symptoms are consistent with a bee sting and she is giving no evidence at this time of anaphylaxis. You should however continue to monitor the patient and urge her to go to the emergency room for a more definitive diagnosis.

34. C

The correct next step is to look for crowning. Answer choice (A) is incorrect, since you have not yet performed an adequate assessment. Answer choice (B) is never correct, as it will endanger both the baby and the mother. (D) is also incorrect, since the only time you place your gloved hand into the birth canal is to assist in maintaining the baby's airway or to loosen the cord if it is wrapped around the baby's neck.

35. B

The correct next action is to prepare for delivery. (A) is incorrect, since with the baby crowning, delivery is now imminent, and you are probably better off in the living room than in the back of the truck. (C) is not going to do any harm, but is not really indicated at this time. (D) is true, but the next thing you must do is open the obstetrical kit and prepare for delivery.

36. A

The correct answer this time is to respond priority to the nearest maternity unit. This is a breech delivery that places the baby at great risk for asphyxia and the mother at risk for delivery complications. The baby has to either be repositioned for a normal vaginal delivery, which is beyond the scope of EMS training, or be delivered by Caesarean section, which is a hospital procedure. You will also want to support the mother with high-flow oxygen and continue to monitor the delivery, and possibly provide airway support to the baby by inserting your hand into the birth canal.

37. B

This patient's violent outburst has no apparent cause and he must be medically evaluated. EMS will always assist police, providing it can be done safely and with a minimum amount of risk to the EMTs. Remember that the police carry weapons and are trained in dealing with violent subjects, whereas EMS is not. (C) is incorrect, since

it could be considered abandonment of a seriously ill patient, and (D) is incorrect, since by removing his handcuffs, he now becomes a danger to the EMTs as well as any other bystanders.

38. B

The patient should be placed in a supine position on a backboard with limbs secured with leather or vinyl cuffs. This position gives the EMT-Basic the best position to continually evaluate the patient and treat any problems as they occur. Answer choice (A) is incorrect, since this patient is at an increased risk for restraint asphyxia. (C) is incorrect because the handcuffs will be forced into the small of his back; also, you will be unable to see the patient or intervene if serious conditions develop. (D) is incorrect because the patient may easily withdraw his limbs and then assault the EMTs.

39. C

The patient's behavior is abnormal and should be considered risky. After you have requested police to respond, you may then take her gently by the arm and escort her to a place where you can evaluate her more thoroughly. (A) is incorrect because her behavior is not violent at this time and she has not demonstrated a clear threat to you, bystanders, or herself. (B) is incorrect because you have not done a thorough examination to determine hypoglycemia. Just because she has had this condition in the past does not mean that this is the case at this time.

40. D

In some jurisdictions, it may be permissible to restrain without medical control. Still, to prevent a future charge of assault, battery, or false imprisonment, it is more prudent to seek medical control. The need to restrain is demonstrated by the patient's attempts to escape from the stretcher; her answers to questions indicate that she is somehow impaired. This patient must be transported to a medical facility for evaluation. Once permission from medical control is obtained, she should be restrained with the least amount of force and restraint necessary. Consequently her wrists could be restrained to the sides of the stretcher, since she is not kicking or punching violently. Handcuffs should not routinely be used by EMS. Answer (C) is technically correct, but probably too intense.

Chapter Seven: **Trauma Emergencies**

- The Golden Hour of Trauma
- Common Traumatic Injuries
- Bleeding and Shock
- Soft Tissue Injuries
- Burns
- Musculoskeletal Care
- Injuries to the Head and Spine
- Injuries to the Eyes, Face, and Neck
- Injuries to the Chest, Abdomen, and Genitalia

THE GOLDEN HOUR OF TRAUMA

Numerous studies have pointed out the survivability of serious trauma patients is substantially higher when surgical intervention is begun within sixty minutes of the injury. Thus the EMT-Basic must calculate the amount of time between the patient's injury and EMS notification, the time spent in responding, the time on scene assessing and treating immediate injuries, and the time that will be required to transport the patient to the trauma center. The goal is getting the patient to the trauma center operating theatre within that "Golden Hour." This will often tax the EMT to use all that he or she has learned with the goal of giving the patient the best possible odds of a successful outcome.

COMMON TRAUMATIC INJURIES

Motor Vehicle Accidents

The most common type of trauma dealt with by EMS is the automobile accident, often dispatched as an "MVA," which stands for Motor Vehicle Accident. Before an EMT-Basic can perform an assessment for a victim of a traumatic injury, he or she must understand how physical forces can cause injury to the human body. This is what is referred to as the kinetics of trauma, or the physics of analyzing the various mechanisms of injury to a body.

If a moving vehicle strikes an immovable object, such as car versus tree, the automobile decelerates from its forward speed to zero, while the driver and passengers continue moving forward at the original rate of speed, striking the interior parts of the car. If the driver is not restrained by a seat belt and the car is moving at fifty miles per hour, he will strike the steering wheel with his chest, abdomen, and pelvis; his head may continue upward into the windshield, which is constructed of double thickness glass with a plastic sheet between the two sheets of glass.

A frontal collision between two moving vehicles is referred to as a head-on collision and the force of impact is the total of both speeds. Thus the damage of a head-on crash of two vehicles doing thirty miles per hour is the equivalent of a single vehicle striking a tree or wall at sixty miles per hour.

A broadside crash in which a vehicle either strikes an object sideways or is struck by another vehicle from the side is referred to as a "T-Bone" crash. Motor vehicle crashes are unique depending on the many factors in play at the time of the crash and the EMT-Basic must be prepared to utilize all of his or her assessment skills in performing a complete patient assessment and treating the resulting multiple injuries.

Falls and Penetration Injuries

Falls are the second most common EMS dispatch for traumatic injury. Again, the EMT must understand how the fall occurred in order to perform a correct assessment. For example, a person who jumps from a second floor window and lands on their feet will be at risk for serious leg and spinal injuries, while a person who falls from the same window and lands face forward will be more at risk for internal organ damage.

Penetration injuries from sharp objects and firearms are a specialty all their own. Urban trauma centers on Friday and Saturday nights are often referred to as "Knife and Gun Clubs" because these type of injuries are brought through their doors.

BLEEDING AND SHOCK

External Bleeding

The average adult human has approximately four quarts of blood in his or her body. If blood is lost as a result of a traumatic injury, the result may be a condition called hypoperfusion syndrome or traumatic shock. This condition is defined as the inadequate circulation of blood through an organ. The sudden loss of one quart of blood from an average adult is considered significant as it affects the circulatory system's ability to perfuse the organs. If blood loss continues, this can lead to shock and death.

There are three types of external bleeding: arterial, venous, and capillary. Arterial bleeding occurs when an artery is lacerated and the blood spurts from the wound. This blood will be bright red as it is oxygen-rich, as opposed to venous blood which is purplish in color because it is oxygen-poor. Arterial bleeding is more difficult to control as it is at a higher pressure. In addition to its darker color, venous bleeding will flow normally rather than spurt from a wound. Capillary bleeding is usually minor and dark red in color and will often clot on its own without outside intervention.

Before an EMT-Basic considers the medical care of external bleeding, he or she must be sure to be wearing the proper protective equipment to assure the EMT's own safety. Depending on the amount of blood involved, this equipment may include disposable gloves, masks, eye protection, and gowns.

Emergency Care of External Bleeding

A patient with a severe amount of bleeding may demand that the EMT immediately stop the loss of blood, but the EMT must always first secure the airway. Remember: a patient without an airway will arrive at the ER dead. After airway is secured, to control external bleeding from an open wound, take a sterile dressing and apply direct pressure to the wound. This will help to constrict the blood flow from the ruptured vessels and promote clotting. Elevation of the wound above the head and torso may also help to slow the flow of blood and help to control the bleeding. If the bleeding cannot be controlled by direct pressure, then more aggressive methods must be taken.

Splinting of a broken bone may help to control bleeding, especially by the use of an air splint. The air splint also holds direct pressure while immobilizing broken bone ends that may be aggravating the wound by lacerating the blood vessel. The use of pressure air splints give the advantage of not only immobilizing the broken bone, but also of applying continuous direct pressure to a wound. These splints may be used to continually apply pressure to a wound even if there is no indication of a fractured bone.

If direct pressure and splinting fail to stop bleeding, pressure to an extremity artery between the heart and the wound may facilitate clotting. These pressure points are where the brachial artery crosses the humerus, the radial artery crosses the wrist, and the femoral artery crosses the femur.

Bleeding from the nose, ears, and mouth may be the result of trauma to the skull and should not be controlled. If the bleeding is a spontaneous epistaxis, or bloody nose, have the patient sit up and lean forward and apply gentle pressure at the bridge of the nose.

Tourniquets

The last resort for controlling bleeding in an extremity is the tourniquet. A tourniquet is a bandage at least four inches wide placed between the heart and the wound as near to the wound as possible.

The tourniquet, when applied and tightened, will stop all blood flow to the wound distal to the device. The consequences of performing this may very well be nerve and tissue damage secondary to the stoppage of oxygenated blood flow to the tissues and cells beyond the application point. Medical control at the receiving facility should be advised immediately that the tourniquet has been applied and "TQ" should be written on the patient's forehead, especially in a mass casualty situation.

To make a tourniquet, tie the bandage with a half hitch and place a stick or bandage scissors on top of the knot, then complete the knot by tying an opposite half hitch to complete a square knot. Twist the stick or scissors to tighten the bandage until the bleeding stops and then secure the stick or scissors with another bandage. A quick tourniquet that can be improvised is the use of the blood pressure cuff; however, it must be carefully monitored for air loss. The tourniquet must always be a wide bandage, never rope or wire that could cut into the tissue and cause necrosis.

Once a tourniquet is applied, it is never loosened, since to do so could result in severe shock as blood rushes from the brain to fill the injured extremity. In addition, a tourniquet should never be applied directly over a joint.

Internal Bleeding

Internal bleeding is more problematic for the EMT since it is not always apparent, yet may lead to severe hypovolemic shock and death. This is especially true when internal organs in the torso have been ruptured due to severe trauma such as an automobile accident or fall. Blunt force trauma can also be caused by blast injuries.

Suspicion of serious internal bleeding may be deduced from the mechanism of injury and signs and symptoms that the EMT finds as he or she performs the trauma assessment. These signs and symptoms would include pain, tenderness, swelling, and discoloration of the suspected site; bleeding from the mouth, rectum, vagina, or other body orifices; blood in vomit, urine, or stool; tenderness, rigidity, and distension of the abdomen.

Treatment of internal bleeding treats the hypoperfusion syndrome that results. Suspicion of internal bleeding will raise the priority of the transport and the "golden hour" becomes much more critical in these types of cases.

Emergency Care of Shock (Hypoperfusion Syndrome)

As the body's own mechanisms respond to attempt to heal and compensate for a traumatic injury, these systems may be overwhelmed. Serious harm may occur as a result of hypoperfusion syndrome or shock. Hemorrhagic shock occurs when the volume of blood becomes insufficient to provide oxygen and nutrients to the cells or remove waste products from the cells. This condition may lead to serious organ damage or death.

The EMT must also be aware of the signs and symptoms of hypovolemic shock which include anxiety or altered mental status, general weakness or dizziness, extreme thirst, tachypnea, tachycardia, skin that is cool, pale, and clammy, capillary refill of longer than two seconds in pediatric patients, nausea and vomiting, and dilated pupils that are sluggish in response to light.

The classic sign of hypovolemic shock is dropping blood pressure. This is considered a late sign and measures for treatment should be begun before it develops. In the case of pediatric patients, since they have a lower blood volume than adults, a dropping blood pressure may indicate that they are close to death, and aggressive treatment is necessary.

Treatment for hypoperfusion syndrome includes the following:
- Maintain the airway, ventilating if necessary
- Administer high flow oxygen
- Control external bleeding
- If your protocols allow, and with the approval of medical control, consider application of a pneumatic antishock garment
- Elevate the lower extremities 8 to 12 inches
- Splint any suspected fractures
- Prevent heat loss by covering the patient with blankets
- Expedite transport to a trauma center as per your protocols.

SOFT TISSUE INJURIES

Before discussing the various types of soft tissue injuries, it is necessary to quickly review the largest organ in the body, the skin. The skin is composed of three layers: the epidermis or outermost layer, the dermis that contains the oil glands and hair follicles, and the subcutaneous layer. The degree of injury will be directly related to how many layers of the skin are involved and treatment protocols will necessitate that the EMT-Basic can recognize these as well.

Closed Injuries

A closed injury is when the epidermis remains intact and there is no external bleeding. There are three types of closed injuries: a contusion or bruise, a hematoma, and a crush injury.
- In a **contusion**, the cells and smaller blood vessels are damaged below the epidermis from some type of trauma and blood pools in the tissues causing a purplish discoloration. This area is often swollen and painful to the touch.

- A **hematoma** involves laceration of a larger blood vessel, either an artery or a vein, and results in a large pool of blood beneath the epidermal layer.
- A **crushing injury** is a closed tissue injury that may cause internal organ rupture; the accompanying bleeding may be so severe as to cause hypoperfusion syndrome (shock).

Emergency medical care for these types of injuries involves appropriate body substance isolation, airway and ventilatory support, treatment for shock, and rapid transport. If the injury involves an extremity, it is often helpful for both treatment of hypovolemia and pain management to splint the extremity. Since these types of injuries cannot be well managed in the prehospital setting, rapid transport to a trauma center is always indicated, remembering the golden hour.

Open Injuries

As opposed to closed injuries, these wounds are open with external bleeding. There are five types of open wounds: abrasions, lacerations, avulsions, penetrations, amputations, and open crushing injuries.

- In an **abrasion**, the epidermal layer is damaged by shearing or scraping. This is a very painful, though superficial injury. While it often generates little blood loss, because of the larger area involved, it is more prone to infection than smaller area wounds.
- In a **laceration**, there is a break in the skin of varying depth; the break may be linear such as in an incision caused by a sharp object or irregular as caused by blunt trauma. Depending on the depth and location, bleeding may be minor to severe. The deeper the wound, the greater the danger of infection as bacteria may have been introduced deep into the tissues by the object causing the laceration.
- An **avulsion** occurs when a flap of skin or tissue is torn off by a traumatic force. These injuries are usually quite painful and will be accompanied by a large volume blood loss.
- A **penetration** or **puncture** wound is a deep intrusion into soft tissue by any object, for example, a bullet or a knife. There may be little or no external bleeding, however the depth of the injury may cause significant internal bleeding. A special consideration in dealing with deep penetration wounds, especially gunshot wounds, is to check for an exit wound, which may be even more pronounced than the entrance wound.
- An **amputation** is the complete separation of a distal extremity or part from the extremity or trunk. Amputations are always traumatic, yet if the amputation is a clean cut rather than a tearing off, bleeding may be minimal.
- **Crushing injuries** may be open or closed and the greater danger is to the underlying organs and tissues.

In the management of these types of injuries, the first concern is to protect the EMT from the dangers of blood-borne pathogens. A massive trauma scenario involving large volumes of blood loss requires more extensive precautions than a simple finger laceration. These precautions may include a full body gown, masks, eye protection, gloves, and shoe coverings. Following treatment of a severe trauma patient, it is always prudent to remain out of service and return to quarters for a shower and change of clothing. Any clothing that has been exposed to blood must be considered contaminated and washed properly, in accordance with local guidelines for dealing with bodily fluid contaminated objects.

Once the scene is safe, including the above-mentioned precautions, it is necessary to secure the patient's airway and provide ventilatory support. In the presence of a gross traumatic injury, EMTs will sometimes focus on the injury site and neglect to check an airway. This is human nature, but always remember that a patient without an airway will arrive at the ER dead.

Once the airway and breathing are secure, the area of bleeding must be exposed and the rest of the body thoroughly checked for other wounds, including exit wounds. If there is arterial bleeding, it must be controlled with direct pressure, elevation, digital pressure, and if necessary, a tourniquet.

With an open wound, prevention of further contamination by bacteria also becomes a concern. Sterile procedures must be used to minimize the danger of further contamination. Once bleeding has been controlled, open wounds should be dressed with dry sterile dressings and secured with clean bandaging materials such as muslin cravats or self-securing bandaging material. Remember that blood loss leads to shock and that the treatment of hypovolemic syndrome must always be a concern.

Special Situations and Treatments

Some wounds due to their location on the body present special situations and require special treatments.

- **Chest wounds, accompanied by a gurgling sound and frothy blood**, indicate that the lung has been penetrated. This may lead to a severely collapsed lung or pneumothorax. If the collapse is so severe as to cause the organs in the chest to shift position, this is referred to as a tension pneumothorax, a life-threatening situation requiring rapid treatment and transport. This type of wound should be dressed with a special sterile dressing, referred to as an occlusive dressing, which will block airflow into the collapsed pleural space. This patient will almost always have compromised breathing and oxygen should always be administered.

- **Abdominal injuries** accompanied by protruding organs, called an **evisceration injury**, are always serious. The wound should be covered with a sterile dressing that has been thoroughly moistened with sterile water or saline. Rapid transport is indicated. The EMT-Basic should not touch the organs or attempt to put them back inside the abdomen.

- **Objects impaled** in the body should not be removed. There are exceptions to this, such as an object through the cheek, an object that would interfere with chest compressions, or an object that would interfere with transport. Medical control is indicated for advice on how to proceed in these situations. The usual treatment is to secure the object as best as possible, control any peripheral bleeding and transport.

- **Extremity amputations** are treated as any other open wound. The amputated part, if possible, should be located and transported along with the patient as it may be possible to reattach it. Wrap the amputated part in a sterile dressing, place it in a plastic bag, and keep it cool by placing the plastic bag on an ice pack. Do not place an amputated part directly on ice as it will freeze. If a part is partly amputated, do not complete the amputation, but stabilize as well as possible.

- **Injuries to the neck that are accompanied by frothy bleeding** may indicate injury to both the airway and blood vessels in the neck. This type of wound should be treated with an occlusive dressing. This will prevent an embolism from entering the circulatory system and causing cardiac or respiratory arrest.

BURNS

Burns are classified according to the depth of the injured tissue. Even though the current literature lists the three categories as superficial, partial thickness, and full thickness, EMTs and hospital staff still refer to these as first, second, and third degree.

- A **first-degree** or **superficial burn** is one that involves only the epidermis and is characterized by a reddening of the skin and local pain. Ordinary sunburn is usually a first-degree burn.
- A **second-degree**, or **partial-thickness burn**, involves both the epidermis and dermis, but does not involve the underlying tissue. It is accompanied by intense pain and blistering of the skin. The skin may be bright red to white.
- A **third-degree** or **full-thickness burn** involves all three layers of skin and may even involve underlying muscles, bones, tissues, and organs. The skin will appear charred, dry, and leathery. Because the sensory nerves have been destroyed or damaged, there may be little or no pain where the skin is burned through, however the peripheral areas will usually have lesser degree burns with extreme pain.

Rule of Nines

The overall survivability of burn injuries is contingent not only upon the type of burn, but on how much of the skin surface is involved. The rule of nines was developed to assist EMS in relaying to the receiving facility how much of the body is involved in the burn injury. There are eleven body areas, each of which contains approximately ninety percent of the body's overall area. They are:

- The head and neck   9 percent
- The chest   9 percent
- The abdomen   9 percent
- The front of each leg (two areas)   18 percent
- The back of each leg (two areas)   18 percent
- The arms (two areas)   18 percent
- The upper back   9 percent
- The lower back   9 percent

These body areas add up to 99 percent; the genitalia comprise the remaining one percent. Thus a patient burned on his face and both arms would be considered to have a burn area of 22 1/2 percent: 9 percent for each arm for a total of 18 and the front of the face for half of nine, or 4.5.

Burn Severity

Burn severity is also gauged by location. Burns to the face and torso are much more problematic due to the danger of inhalation of the products of combustion, making swelling to the airway and fluid buildup in the lungs possible. Once the type of burn and the area of body surface affected has been determined, the EMT-Basic can determine the severity of the injury.

The following burn conditions are considered to be a critical injury and should be expedited:

- Any third-degree burns that involve the hands, feet, face, or genitalia
- Any burn that may involve respiratory damage
- Full-thickness burns involving more than 10 percent of the body surface
- Partial-thickness burns involving more than 30 percent of the body surface
- Any burns complicated by painful, swollen, or deformed extremities
- Moderate burns to pediatric and geriatric patients
- Any burns which encompass an entire body part, such as an arm, leg, chest, etc.

A moderate-burn injury is considered to be:

- Any full-thickness burn involving 2 to 10 percent of the body area unless it involves the hands, feet, face, genitalia, or upper chest
- Any partial-thickness burn involving 15 to 30 percent of the body area
- Any first-degree burn involving more than 50 percent of the body surface.

Using this criterion, a male who has a sunburn which covers all of his body except beneath the area covered by a bathing suit has a superficial burn covering between 70 to 80 percent of his body area and this would be considered a moderate burn injury, not a minor burn.

A minor burn is:

- A superficial burn covering less than 50 percent of the body's surface
- A partial-thickness burn covering less than 15 percent of the body's area
- A full-thickness burn covering less than two percent of the body's area.

Emergency Care of Burns

Emergency medical care of burn patients involves stopping the burning process. This is initially accomplished by copious application of water or saline solution to the burnt area following the removal of burnt clothing and any jewelry. The EMT-Basic must be especially alert for airway compromise if the airway has been exposed in any way to products of combustion. Infection is also a prime consideration in management of burn victims, so extreme caution should be used in order to create as sterile an environment for the patient as possible. Burnt areas, once cooled, should be covered with loose sterile dressings. To minimize the risk of infection, blisters should never be broken and ointments, lotions, or antiseptics should never be applied in the emergency care scenario.

Chemical burns should be neutralized by flushing with water or with fluids recommended for a particular chemical by the label or manufacturer's safety data sheet. Dry chemical caustic powders should be brushed off the skin before flushing and care must be taken not to allow the runoff fluid from washing to injure unaffected body parts.

Electrical burns are a concern for the safety of the responding crew. The EMT-Basic must be sure that the person is still not energized by contact with the electrical object that caused the injury. If unsure, do not touch the patient out of concern for your own safety. Once you have determined that the patient is safe to touch, treat the wound as you would any burn. On assessment, be aware that contact with an electrical object may result in both an entrance wound and an exit wound as the electricity goes to ground. Also, electrocution may cause cardiac dysrhythmias. It is appropriate to monitor an electrocution victim with an AED to assure that electrocountershock is readily available in the event that the victim's heart begins to fibrillate.

MUSCULOSKELETAL CARE

Injuries to the musculoskeletal system of the body are among the most challenging to the EMT-Basic. The principles of this type of care are important to understand since trauma patients will rarely present with a textbook example of a musculoskeletal injury. The EMT-Basic will have to improvise treatment utilizing these principles.

In order to implement a treatment plan for these injuries, a study of the mechanism of injury (MOI) is necessary. The NREMT curriculum mentions three types of force that cause injury: direct force, indirect force, and twisting force.

- In **direct force**, the injury occurs at the point of impact. If a window falls onto someone's forearm and fractures the radius, this is an example of a direct force injury.
- In **indirect force**, the injury occurs away from the point of impact. An example of indirect force would be when a subject falls and lands on his feet and the force of the landing causes his hip to dislocate.
- **Twisting force**, as the name implies, occurs when one part of an extremity remains stationary while another part rotates. The best example of this is a sprained ankle.

There are two types of bone and joint injuries, open and closed. Simply put, a broken bone or torn tissue with a break in the continuity of the skin is called an open fracture, sprain, or strain. If there is no break in the skin, then it is a closed fracture, sprain, or strain. An open fracture is a combination injury that requires treatment of the broken bone or damaged joint and management of the accompanying wound.

The signs and symptoms of a bone or joint injury are: deformity, pain, grating, swelling, discoloration, exposed bone ends, or locked joint. Emergency care is to splint the injury, apply cold to reduce swelling, and elevate the extremity to reduce the pain, as well as treat for shock.

Splinting

Management of musculoskeletal injuries involves a science known as splinting. Simply put, splinting is immobilizing a broken bone or damaged joint, as well as any adjacent joints. A properly applied splint will help to prevent further damage to tissues irritated by the broken bone ends. Splinting will also minimize the danger that a closed injury may progress to an open injury, further complicating patient care and resulting in a much longer recovery period.

Prior to applying a splint, distal pulse, motor, and sensation must be assessed in order to compare these vital signs once the splint has been applied. The splint must immobilize the area where the EMT-Basic suspects the break has occurred, as well as the adjacent joints. A suspected mid-shaft tibia fracture must not only immobilize the mid-shaft area of the bone, but also the ankle joint and knee joint.

Prior to application of any splint, clothing must be removed or cut away. In the case of the lower extremities, shoes and boots must be removed to assure proper application of a splint and as well as assessment of distal neural vital signs. If the fracture is open, the wounds must be dressed with a sterile dressing prior to splint application. If the extremity is severely deformed or if the distal area is cyanotic and pulses and sensation are absent, than the limb must be realigned with gentle traction prior to splinting.

Types of Splints

There are many different types of splints, including improvised splints used in Wilderness EMS. Basically, a splint is any object that immobilizes the suspected injury and adjacent joints. The splints most common to EMS are the rigid board splints, which come in a variety of sizes. These boards are then secured in whatever configuration is necessary with the use of cravats or straps. Variations of these include the vinyl splints with rigid spines that secure quickly with Velcro™. A long spineboard is an example of a board splint that can immobilize the entire body. Many EMT-Basics prefer the use of vacuum or air pressure splints, which in addition to splinting also provide pressure uniformly to the extremity, often useful in wound management as well. The PASG is a type of air splint that also immobilizes the entire lower body, including the pelvis. The traction splint is a special type of splint that provides continuous traction of the lower extremities and is often indicated by protocol for management of closed femur fractures. Likewise, many ordinary objects can be adapted for splinting, such as pillows and large magazines.

Traction Splints

A traction splint is a special device that not only immobilizes the broken bone, but also alleviates pain by applying continuous traction to keep the broken bone ends from further aggravating the tissue in the extremity. Its use is governed by local protocol and is usually limited to suspected closed mid-shaft femur fractures.

The application of the traction splint is required as a practical skill by most EMS courses (see pages 145–147 for photos). The proper application of the traction splint is accomplished by first checking for distal pulses and neurological response. The EMT-Basic then places the ankle strap of the device around the patient's ankle and applies gentle traction by pulling on the ankle hitch while supporting the lower leg with the other hand. An assistant then takes traction so that the EMT-Basic can apply the traction device. The length of the device is set by using the uninjured leg as a guide, with the traction winch six to eight inches beyond the bottom of the foot. Moving the splint next to the injured leg on the lateral side, the EMT-Basic palpates for the pelvic ischium (the floor of the pelvis) and places the superior end of the splint against it. The strap of the splint is then secured around the leg, holding the splint firmly against the pelvis. The EMT-Basic then hooks the ankle hitch to the winch and applies mechanical traction, taking traction over from the assistant. Using the uninjured leg as a guide, the EMT-Basic continues to apply traction until the injured leg is slightly longer, or until the patient feels that the pain is lessening at the site of the suspected fracture. The support straps of the splint are then wrapped around the leg, avoiding the site of the injury and the knee. Distal neurological signs are again checked and noted, and the patient is now ready to be placed on a spineboard for transport.

Once a splint has been applied, it is imperative that the distal neural vital signs be checked again as it is possible to cut off blood supply to the distal extremity with an improperly applied splint. This can result in tissue damage and even in the necessity of amputating the distal portion of the extremity. Also the time taken to splint an obvious or suspected injury may delay life-saving treatment for other conditions at the hospital. Many times an unstable patient (such as a patient with an airway injury) is secured quickly to a backboard (the all-purpose universal splint) and transported priority with all other assessments and treatments done en route.

INJURIES TO THE HEAD AND SPINE

The brain is the organ that is responsible for operating the multiple systems of the human body by receiving sensory information and sending electrical impulses to the organs, muscles, and tissues via the nervous system. The spinal cord that runs from the base of the brain down the back is the main transmission line for these actions and if it is damaged or severed as a result of trauma, then these systems may be compromised. The spinal cord is surrounded and protected by the bony spinal column, which is composed of 33 bones called vertebrae.

EMT-Basics will be assisted in their assessment of these types of injuries if they pay close attention to the mechanism of injury and picture what may have happened to the body of the patient as a result of these forces. The spinal cord may be compressed if the patient has been in a situation where significant force has been applied to the top of the head. Someone who dives head first into an empty swimming pool and strikes the bottom is an example of this type of injury. The spinal column and cord may also be damaged by excessive motion (for example, in sports injuries). The spinal column may also be distracted by excessive stretching (hanging by the neck, for example).

Spinal Injuries

As the EMT-Basic performs the assessment, the suspicion of a spinal cord injury rises significantly if any of the following signs or symptoms are present: tenderness or pain in the back or neck; pain when the neck or back is moved; intermittent pain in the spinal column or legs independent of motion or palpation; any open injuries to the back or neck; numbness, tingling, or weakness in the extremities; loss of sensation or motion in the extremities; incontinence.

If a spinal injury is suspected and the patient is responsive, it is imperative to ask the patient if he or she has back or neck pain, if he or she can move his or her fingers and toes without pain, and if he or she can feel the EMT-Basic touching his or her extremities. Following inspection and palpation of the neck, back, and extremities, and as part of the focused trauma assessment, the EMT-Basic asks the patient to grab his or her hands and squeeze as hard as he or she can to determine if there is a difference in grip strength and if this reflex causes pain. The EMT-Basic then pushes gently on the soles of the patient's feet and asks the patient to push down, again with the goal of ascertaining if there is equal strength in the lower extremities. If the spinal cord injury is located in the cervical vertebrae, then the ability to breathe or move the extremities may be compromised and the EMT-Basic must be prepared to intervene to correct these conditions.

In case of a possible injury, the spinal cord must be immobilized in a neutral (straight) position. To do this, take the head in both hands and hold it gently so that it is aligned with the spine. The EMT-Basic can also use the first and middle fingers to perform a modified jaw thrust to secure a patent airway. This stabilization must be maintained until the patient is secured to a spineboard. Once the patient is secured in this manner and has a patent airway, is breathing, has a palpable carotid pulse, and has no gross hemorrhage, then the remainder of the initial assessment can be performed.

Once the head and neck have been assessed by sight and touch, a rigid cervical collar should be applied to assist with maintaining stabilization. A rigid cervical collar must be the correct size for the patient and must be properly applied or more harm can result. The collar must hold the head and chin up in the neutral position without hyperextending the neck. The collar must touch the skin on the chest and back, as well as the chin and back of the neck.

Securing to a Spineboard

Once the initial assessment is complete, the patient is then secured to a spineboard (see photos on pages 142–144). To do this, one EMT places the board next to the patient. Three people should kneel on the opposite side of the patient with their arms over the patient and their hands below the patient. The person holding the head then assures that everyone is ready and on the count of three, the people roll the patient on his or her side towards them as the person holding the head rolls the head with them keeping the head aligned with the spine. One EMT quickly assesses the posterior side of the patient and then the EMT controlling the spineboard places it beneath the patient's side. Once everyone is again in position and ready, the EMT holding the head again counts to three and on three the patient is rolled again to the supine position, this time on the spineboard. The patient is then properly positioned on the board at the command of the EMT holding cervical stabilization. The patient is then secured to the board using a minimum of three straps, one across the chest, one across the pelvis, and one across the legs. The head is then secured to the board using an approved device, usually head blocks and Velcro™ straps. All distal neurological signs are again checked and the patient, now properly splinted, is removed to the truck for transport.

If the patient with a suspected neck or spinal injury is found in a sitting position, a short spineboard or intermediate transport device such as a Kendrick Extrication Device (see photos on pages 139–141) is used to remove the victim from the immediate area to a long spineboard.

Head Injuries

Injuries to the head present a special challenge to the EMT-Basic. The scalp is extremely vascular and any open wound will cause a large amount of bleeding. In addition, even a closed wound from blunt force trauma may cause bleeding inside the cranial compartment, causing increasing pressure inside the skull and complicating breathing and circulation. In addition to trauma, some medical conditions, such as stroke, may give the same signs and symptoms as head trauma.

The EMT-Basic should suspect a brain injury when any of the following are present during the primary or focused assessment: altered or decreasing mental status; irregular breathing; bleeding or bruising to the head; blood or fluid (cerebrospinal fluid) leading from the ears, eyes, nose, or mouth; bruising around the eyes (raccoon eyes); bruising behind the ears (Battle's sign); any neurological disability; nausea and vomiting; pupils of different sizes with altered mental status; seizure activity.

Treatment of Suspected Skull Fracture or Brain Injury

For these conditions, the decision to expedite transport is imperative since the patient must be seen in a trauma center with appropriate equipment as soon as possible. Any head injury is assumed to involve the cervical spine, so head and spinal immobilization are always indicated. Closely monitor the patient for abrupt changes in mental status and vital signs and intervene as appropriate. Bleeding from the head should be controlled as any open wound, however, do not apply pressure to an open or depressed skull wound, since there is the danger of pushing a bone fragment into the brain or increasing the intercranial pressure.

Special considerations for dealing with head or spinal injuries include the decision to extricate the patient from his or her situation using the time consuming method of full spinal and head immobilization, or to rapidly extricate the patient using minimal immobilization. Situations that would necessitate rapid immobilization include: an unsafe environment, such as the potential for fire or explosion; a patient who is unstable, i.e. not breathing or with no circulation; the patient's position is blocking access to a more critically injured patient.

Another special consideration in head and spine injuries is the removal of a sports or motorcycle helmet. Current protocols advise that unless it is necessary to ventilate a patient or treat a severe bleeding wound, the helmet should be left on and spinal stabilization be performed with the helmet in place. Face guards and shields are easily removed for assessment and should be accomplished rapidly.

If it is necessary to remove a helmet, it should be done quickly. One EMT should be stabilizing the head and neck as the second EMT spreads the helmet as wide as possible and then pushes it upwards attempting to minimize the movement and strain on the head and neck. Again, it should only be removed if a potentially life-threatening condition exists that needs intervention in the field.

INJURIES TO THE EYES, FACE, AND NECK

Eye Injuries

Injuries to the eye are always considered serious since they may have long-term consequences to the quality of life of a victim of trauma. In assessing trauma to the eyes, in addition to palpating for broken bones, the EMT-Basic should use his or her diagnostic penlight to determine the reactivity of the pupils to light and compare the responses from each eye to the other. Also the patient should be able to track the light with his or her eyes without moving the head and the tracking should be smooth for both eyes.

Often foreign objects will take up residence in the eye. Small particles of dust and other foreign matter are usually removed by flushing the eyeball with sterile water or saline. Chemicals and irritants splashed into the eyes can also be removed by flushing. One method for maintaining continuous flushing is to place a nasal oxygen cannula connected to an IV set and a 1 liter bag of saline instead of oxygen. The cannula should be over the bridge of the nose with the nasal prongs resting over the medial edge of the eye socket.

If there is a penetrating injury to the eye, the object is not removed, but secured in place with bandages and dressings. In this type of injury to the eye, both eyes are always covered so that the parallel motion of the uninjured eye does not cause the injured eye to move. In the case of an avulsed eyeball, do not attempt to replace the eye, but cover the eyeball with a clean paper cup and bandage it in place to protect the eye.

Face Injuries

Injuries to the face are treated in the same way as other injuries with the exception that an impaled object through the cheek may be removed by the EMT-Basic in the field in order to facilitate management of the airway. Remember that because of the extensive vasculature of the face and head, injuries to these areas will bleed profusely.

Neck Injuries

Injuries to the neck may involve the great vessels leading the brain, as well as injury to the airway. Bubbling and gurgling of a neck wound are indications that the injury not only involves the blood vessels, but also the airway. This type of wound requires an occlusive dressing to prevent outside air from entering the blood vessel and causing an air embolism.

INJURIES TO THE CHEST, ABDOMEN, AND GENITALIA

Chest Injuries

If the assessment of a trauma victim reveals paradoxical motion of the rib cage, combined with pain and crepitis of the ribs, this is an indication of a condition called flail chest, defined as two or more ribs broken in two or more places. The paradoxical motion, or area that falls when the chest rises and rises when chest falls, is caused by the broken or flailed area floating freely on the chest wall. This type of injury must be splinted to the application of an IV bag, sandbag, or similar object to the flail area, and bandaged in place to minimize the paradoxical motion.

Chest injuries that are bubbling are called "sucking chest wounds" and, like neck wounds, must be dressed with an occlusive dressing to prevent air from entering the pleural space and increasing the likelihood of a pneumothorax. These occlusive dressings may be waterproof thin-film-type dressings, or lubricated gauze pads. In an emergency, commercial plastic wrap can also be used.

Closed chest wounds are especially dangerous, especially if they involve the heart or the great vessels leading to and from the heart. A serious condition known as cardiac tamponade, caused by blunt trauma to the heart, occurs when the sac around the heart (pericardium) fills with blood and places pressure on the heart. Since there is no basic intervention that can be done in the field, if the EMT-Basic suspects this type of injury, the patient is a load and go. The EMT-Basic should be especially alert for trauma patients who spit or cough up blood as these patients have a higher suspicion of a closed chest injury involving the heart or lungs.

Abdominal Injuries

Abdominal injuries place patients at an increased risk of infection of the abdominal cavity if the hollow organs of the digestive system become ruptured and discharge the digestive products into the peritoneal space. Rigidity and tenderness of the abdomen are indications of this and transport should be expedited.

If the injury has exposed the intestines and they are protruding from the wound, the EMT-Basic should not attempt to replace them, but they should be dressed with sterile dressings and irrigated with sterile water or saline.

Injuries to the Genitalia

Injuries to the genitalia in both males and females are extremely painful due to the high concentration of nerves in this area. Injuries to these areas are treated in the same way as any other wounds.

A special consideration with male genitalia is a condition known as testicular tortion, which is caused when a testicle becomes twisted in the scrotum, causing severe pain. This injury is caused by strenuous activity and must be corrected in the emergency room. Emergency care consists of application of an ice pack to relieve the pain and careful transport to minimize movement.

Victims of sexual assault require special handling by the emergency medical system, since EMTs are often the first responders to these occurrences. Most states require medical personnel to report these events to the police, especially if the victim is a minor. The EMT-Basic must be careful to preserve any evidence of a crime, such as torn clothing and stains from blood and other fluids. In dealing with the victims, it is almost always better to have the victim assessed by an EMT of the same gender if possible. Care should be supportive and affirming, without making unrealistic promises. Sexual assault victims are often sensitive to being touched in any way by an EMT, so explanations in a calm voice are necessary. Remember that a patient, unless impaired or unconscious, has the right to refuse any medical procedure, so request the patient's permission to perform each and every assessment, particularly those involving the genitals.

PRACTICE SET

1. You are dispatched to a motorcycle accident on the Interstate. You respond priority and arrive on the scene ten minutes after being dispatched. Your patient is unconscious and unresponsive to any stimuli. Your rapid assessment shows that he is breathing with ragged breaths at a rate of 16, has a pulse of 60 with a pulse oximetry of 94 percent. He is lying 80 feet from his motorcycle face down on the pavement. Your transport time to the trauma center is thirty minutes. How long do you have to assess and treat this patient on the scene?

   (A) 10 minutes

   (B) 20 minutes

   (C) 30 minutes

   (D) Enough time to properly treat all of the patient's injuries

2. Two vehicles collide, head on, on a busy highway. The speed limit is 50 mph. What is your estimated speed of impact?

   (A) 50 mph

   (B) 70 mph

   (C) 90 mph

   (D) 100 mph

3. You are dispatched to a two car motor vehicle accident on a rural highway. You arrive on scene and the incident commander directs you to a car that has been struck broadside by the other vehicle. There is severe damage to the driver's side of the vehicle and the driver is lying on the front seat on his back. He is unconscious and unresponsive. He appears pale and diaphoretic with a weak thready pulse. His right leg is lying beneath the steering wheel at an awkward angle. He has a large scalp laceration which is bleeding purplish blood. You are wearing suitable precautions against blood-borne pathogens. Which of the following is the next correct step in the management of this patient?

   (A) Gently splint the right leg with a board splint

   (B) Apply a sterile dressing to the scalp laceration

   (C) Perform a rapid extrication and transport priority to the trauma center

   (D) Take cervical stabilization and open the airway using the modified jaw thrust

4. In the scenario in question 3, your patient is breathing at a rate of 24 times per minute and has a pulse of 80. What would be your next treatment?

   (A) Gently splint the right leg with a board splint

   (B) Apply a sterile dressing to the scalp laceration

   (C) Perform a rapid extrication and transport priority to the trauma center

   (D) Apply a cervical collar and maintain stabilization of the head and neck

5. In the scenario described in question 3, your patient has been extricated to the truck on a spineboard with full cervical stabilization. The right leg has been splinted and the head wound is dressed. Your assessment of the head reveals nothing unremarkable and as you examine his chest you notice a large bruise on the right side of his chest. His blood pressure is 95/65. Which of the following is NOT a treatment for hypovolemic shock?

   (A) Elevate the foot of the spineboard 8 to 12 inches

   (B) Warm the patient with blankets

   (C) Elevate the head of the spineboard 8 to 12 inches

   (D) Administer high flow oxygen via NRB mask at 12 lpm

6. In the scenario described in question 3, your response time to the scene was 10 minutes. You now estimate it will take you 15 minutes to transport your patient to the trauma center. How many minutes should you spend triaging and treating your patient on scene?

   (A) Ten minutes

   (B) Twenty minutes

   (C) Thirty minutes

   (D) As long as it takes

7. Which of the following cannot be used to control severe bleeding?

   (A) Tourniquet

   (B) Sterile gauze pad

   (C) Air splint

   (D) Oxygen mask

8. You respond to a fight in progress call to assist police with a possible gunshot victim. You arrive on scene wearing suitable protective equipment and the police have secured the scene. They direct you to a male in his mid twenties, lying supine on the ground. His shirt is full of blood and he is conscious and alert, but having trouble breathing. What should be your next move?

   (A) Apply a tourniquet to both arms to minimize extremity blood flow

   (B) Apply a non-rebreather mask and administer oxygen at 12 liters per minute

   (C) Remove the shirt and check for wounds

   (D) Place the patient on a backboard and transport immediately to the nearest trauma center

9. In the scenario in question 8, you observe a puncture wound 1/2 inch in diameter in the left chest 2 inches superior to the left nipple. It is actively bleeding bright red frothy blood. What is your next procedure?

   (A) Apply sterile 4 x 4 gauze dressing to the wound

   (B) Apply sterile occlusive dressing

   (C) Apply a trauma dressing

   (D) Request an ALS intercept

10. In the scenario in question 8, what is the thing that you will have to be especially alert for as you continue your focused assessment?

   (A) Patient's legal status

   (B) Patient's blood pressure

   (C) Patient's lung sounds

   (D) The exit wound

11. How do you treat an amputated finger?

   (A) Transport it with the patient.

   (B) Secure it to the patient's hand with sterile gauze and tape.

   (C) Keep it cool by placing it directly on an ice pack.

   (D) Transport it separately in a second rescue or police car to avoid traumatizing the patient.

12. Which of the following impaled objects should you remove in the field?

    (A) Pencil through the cheek

    (B) Fishing spear imbedded in the left thigh

    (C) Fence post through the abdomen

    (D) Knife embedded in the chest causing a pneumothorax

13. You respond to a house explosion with fire and police. You have suitable protective equipment and the scene is secure upon your arrival. On scene you are directed to a patient with soot on his face. The patient states rather sheepishly that he was lighting his charcoal grill and, having run out of lighter fluid, poured gasoline on the charcoal and then attempted to light it, resulting in an explosion. He is conscious and alert with first-degree burns to both his arms and hands and his face. What is your primary concern with this patient?

    (A) Anaphylactic shock

    (B) Danger of infection

    (C) Airway compromise

    (D) Secondary explosion

14. In the scenario in question13, approximately what percentage of the patient's body is burnt?

    (A) 10 percent

    (B) 20 percent

    (C) 30 percent

    (D) 40 percent

15. In the scenario in questions 13 and 14, what is the severity of this patient?

    (A) Critical

    (B) Moderate

    (C) Minor

    (D) Fatal

16. You respond to an industrial plant for an injured worker. You respond priority with suitable BSI precautions. You arrive on scene and observe a male lying atop a wire, obviously unconscious. Which of the following should be your primary concern?

    (A) Airway

    (B) Scene safety

    (C) Burn injury

    (D) Cardiac dysrhythmias

17. You arrive on the scene of a motorcycle accident, the police are on scene, and you are wearing suitable BSI gear. The driver is lying supine fifteen feet away from his motorcycle which is lying on its side. He is screaming in pain and you perform your initial assessment and rapid trauma assessment. He is conscious, alert, and oriented with no injuries other than an angulated right femur which is causing him severe pain. His vitals are BP 160/100, pulse is 120, and respirations are 22. Which of the following devices should you use to splint his injury?

    (A) PASG

    (B) Traction splint

    (C) Long spineboard

    (D) Inflatable splint

18. You respond to a soccer field for an injured player. You respond priority wearing suitable precautions. When you arrive on the scene you are directed to the soccer field where an eleven-year-old female is conscious, alert, and oriented, lying supine in severe pain. She is clutching her left upper arm with her right hand and her shoulder is displaced to the anterior. Bystanders state she was in a collision with another player and fell to the ground. She did not lose consciousness, her vital signs are within normal limits, and the remainder of the assessment is unremarkable. What injury do you suspect?

    (A) Broken humerus

    (B) Broken radius

    (C) Dislocated patella

    (D) Dislocated shoulder

19. In the scenario in question 18, what device are you going to use to splint this injury?

    (A) Full arm air splint

    (B) Full arm board splint

    (C) Tourniquet

    (D) Backboard and padding

20. A splint should NOT be applied to which of the following:

    (A) Suspected fractures

    (B) Suspected strains

    (C) Suspected sprains

    (D) Suspected hemothorax

21. You are dispatched to a man fallen off a ladder at his home. You arrive on the scene with suitable BSI precautions and find a male sitting on the floor with a blood-soaked trouser leg. He is conscious, alert, and oriented, has normal vital signs, and no other injuries or loss of consciousness. You expose the leg by gently cutting the trouser leg away and observe that the fibula is broken and the superior end is exposed through the anterior side of the leg. What must you do BEFORE you splint the leg?

    (A) DCAP-BTLS

    (B) Request medical control for permission to splint

    (C) Apply a sterile dressing to the wound

    (D) Irrigate the wound with sterile saline

22. In the scenario in question 21, the patient had a good pedal pulse prior to your applying the splint. Upon rechecking, it is no longer palpable and the foot is becoming cold and cyanotic. You should next

    (A) Request an ALS intercept

    (B) Remove the splint

    (C) Expedite the transport

    (D) Immobilize the patient on a spineboard

23. You arrive on the scene of a two car motor vehicle accident and the incident commander directs you to the first car which was rear ended by the second car. The driver is alone in the vehicle and is still wearing his seat belt. He is conscious, alert, and oriented, and is complaining of neck pain and being unable to turn his head. You and your partner are wearing appropriate BSI gear and there is no gross hemorrhage. What should be your next move?

    (A) Rapidly extricate onto a long spineboard

    (B) Place on a short spineboard and extricate

    (C) Take manual stabilization from the rear seat and apply a cervical collar

    (D) Perform a modified jaw thrust

24. In the scenario in question 23, what would be the correct next action if the car was on fire?

    (A) Rapidly extricate onto a long spineboard

    (B) Place on a short spineboard and extricate

    (C) Take manual stabilization from the rear seat and apply a cervical collar

    (D) Perform a modified jaw thrust

25. You are dispatched to a home under construction for a man fallen off a roof. You respond priority and arrive on scene. Your patient is a roofer who walked off the roof and fell approximately twenty feet to the ground. He is conscious, but dazed. He has an airway, his respiratory rate is 14, and his pulse is 72. There is no gross hemorrhage or sign of any bleeding. Your partner takes manual stabilization of the head and neck while you perform a rapid trauma assessment, which is negative for any potentially broken bones. You apply a cervical collar and log roll him onto a spineboard and secure him. En route to the trauma center you expose the patient by cutting of his clothes and your focused exam is negative, however when you push against his feet he complains of pain in the back of his neck. What injury should you suspect?

    (A) Ruptured spleen
    (B) Broken femur
    (C) Fractured cervical vertebra
    (D) Fractured skull

26. You respond to the local high school football field on a Saturday afternoon for an injured player. You arrive on scene with the correct BSI gear and are directed to midfield where an 18-year-old male wearing a helmet is lying on his back. He is unconscious and not responsive to your questioning. You are unable to perform an airway maneuver or to ascertain his respirations. Your next move is to:

    (A) Perform a modified jaw thrust
    (B) Attempt to insert an oropharyngeal airway
    (C) Stabilize his head and neck and remove the helmet
    (D) Secure the helmet on a spineboard and expedite transport

ANSWER EXPLANATIONS

1. A

In reading the question, you may be tempted to take the 60 minutes of the Golden Hour, subtract the 10 minute response time and the 30 minute hospital transport time and arrive at 20 minutes, but this does not factor in the amount of time that transpired before you were dispatched. This will be the sum of the minutes spent until someone finds the patient, dials and is connected to the dispatch center, and the lag time while dispatch processes the incoming information and dispatches your unit. This amount of time is a variable and is dependent on a number of factors. In addition, once you arrive at the trauma center, medical personnel will triage the patient and stabilize him in the emergency room before sending him to the operating suite, which will add more minutes. (D) is a tempting answer and may sound logically correct, but if you properly treat all of these injuries on the scene, you will definitely exceed the Golden Hour.

2. D

In a head on crash impact speed is the combined speed of both vehicles and the injuries would be consistent if one vehicle had crashed into a wall at that speed.

3. D

The temptation is always to treat the most noticeable condition first, such as the active bleeding or the obvious fracture. However, you first and foremost must be concerned with the patient's survival; without an airway, he will be dead in minutes. In addition, the patient's cervical spine must be stabilized prior to any other treatments to minimize the danger of damaging the spinal cord. Answer (D) takes care of both those things and must be the priority in this scenario.

4. D

The correct answer is apply a cervical collar and stabilize. There is no indication that a rapid extrication is indicated. There is a temptation to treat the obvious head wound, but since the bleeding is purplish and nonpulsing, it is probably venous and can be controlled once your patient is better stabilized and extricated.

5. C

The correct answer is (C) in this tricky NOT question. The others are all correct treatments of hypovolemic shock. Don't get confused between the apparent similarity of answer choices (A) and (C), since in the former you are elevating the foot of the spineboard, not the head..

6. A

The correct answer is 10 minutes. Twenty minutes will still be under the one hour guide, but does not take into account discovery and notification time, nor triage time at the hospital. Thirty minutes will obviously put you over the hour, as would the impossible EMT luxury of "taking as long as you like." This scene is managed by quickly performing the procedures necessary to save the patient's life and packaging him for transport. Further assessments and treatments may be accomplished en route.

7. D

An oxygen mask may be indicated for help in treating hypovolemic shock, however, it is not directly used to control severe bleeding. The other choices all are methods of controlling severe bleeding.

8. C

You need to visualize what you're dealing to be able to intervene properly. Applying a tourniquet to minimize extremity blood flow is not an acceptable procedure for any injury. You may well want to administer supplemental oxygen after you've done a proper assessment, but the assessment is the important thing at this stage, likewise is the expedited transport.

9. B

The correct next procedure is to apply a sterile occlusive dressing. Answers (A) and (C) will do nothing to seal the opening in the pleural space that air is escaping from, which is what is causing the frothy blood. The danger here is that this patient will develop a tension pneumothorax or hemothorax. You may request an ALS intercept to assist with advanced life support measures; however, you would do this after you have taken care of the life-threatening conditions, such as the gross hemorrhage.

10. D

In gunshot cases, there is often an exit wound which can be easily overlooked if the assessment is not as thorough as it should be. The patient's legal status, i.e. whether or not he is in police custody, should have no bearing on your interventions. The patient's blood pressure and lung sounds are important as well, but are part of usual assessments. What you would need to be "especially alert" for in the case of a puncture wound is an exit wound.

11. D

The amputated extremity should be wrapped in a sterile wet dressing, placed in a cool container, and transported with the patient to the appropriate facility. Attempting to secure it to the patient's hand with gauze and tape will only delay transport and not have any long-term benefit. Placing it directly on an ice pack could cause it to freeze and the tissue to die. There is no reason to transport it separately either.

12. A

The correct answer is (A), because a pencil through the cheek will interfere with respiration. The other answers will not impede the airway and should be left for the emergency room to deal with.

13. C

The correct answer is airway compromise. The nature of the explosion and the fact that his face is burnt gives him a high probability that he inhaled the flame and smoke from the explosion. Anaphylactic shock is the result of an allergic reaction and the danger of infection is less problematic than the risk of his airway swelling shut. A secondary explosion has hopefully been minimized by the fire department's securing of the scene.

14. B

Using the rule of nines, each arm counts for 9 percent for a total of 18. The whole head is 9 percent, but in this case, only the face is involved and counts for 4.5 percent. This gives a total of 22.5 percent and answer choice (B) is the closest.

15. A

This is a critical patient because of the danger of airway compromise due to burns to his face. The patient could also be considered critical simply because two entire body parts, the arms, are involved. Some test takers may answer "moderate" incorrectly because they base their answer only by the percentage of body area affected, which is less than the 50 percent necessary for this burn to be considered critical if there were no other factors.

16. B

The correct answer is scene safety. All of the other answer choices become concerns once you have determined that the patient is not being energized by the wire he is lying across.

17. B

While any of the devices listed may be used, the traction splint is the preferred device for this injury.

18. D

It is important to read the question and get a picture of what the questioner is describing. You could stop with the upper arm and deduce that the correct answer is the broken humerus, but the anterior displacement of the shoulder is key that this is a dislocation or fracture of the shoulder joint.

19. D

A backboard is the only device listed which will immobilize the entire joint. (A) and (B) are devices which will only immobilize the arm and elbow joint. (C) is used for controlling bleeding in extreme necessity.

20. D

Since it is impossible to definitely diagnose these conditions in the field, all bone and joint injuries must be splinted. A hemothorax is a pleural space that is filling with blood and does not call for a splint.

21. C

This is a combination of an open wound and a fracture and both must be treated. You will already have done DCAP-BTLS and most systems do not require the EMT-Basic to secure medical control to apply splints. Irrigation of the wound may or may not be advisable due to a number of conditions, which is why (C) is the best answer.

22. B

In applying the splint you may have occluded an artery supplying blood to the foot. The other answers are all possibilities, but you have to correct the problem caused by applying the splint.

23. C

The patient is talking to you so you know that there is an airway and that the patient is breathing. Before extricating him from the vehicle your next priority is to secure the head and neck. Once that is accomplished, the next step would be to place him on a short spineboard and extricate. There is no indication in the question that the scene is unstable, which would then require a rapid extrication.

24. A

Rapid extrication is now necessary due to the danger of further injury to you and the patient in the now unstable scene.

25. C

Pain to the neck as you are applying pressure to the soles of the feet indicates some type of pressure to the spinal cord. All of the other injuries are possible given the MOI, however there is nothing in the question to indicate that any of these are the correct answer.

26. C

If this patient is not breathing and does not have a patent airway, he will die before you can get him to a hospital. The airway and ventilation support take priority over any other protocols and you must get access to his mouth and nose to perform the necessary airway interventions.

APPLICATION OF THE KENDRICK EXTRICATION DEVICE

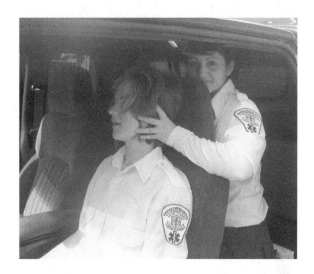

1. The EMT-Basic must first take manual stabilization of the cervical spine and indicate to the examiner that it is secure.

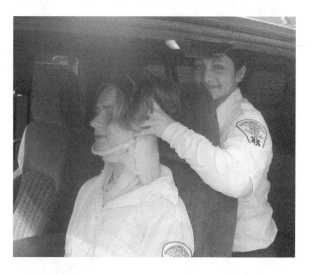

2. The EMT-Basic must then pass off stabilization to a partner without compromising constant stability and correctly size and apply a cervical collar.

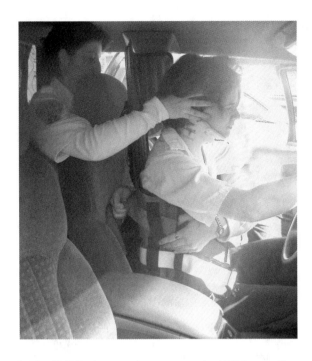

3. The EMT-Basic must then prepare the KED for application and center the device in place behind the patient with a minimum of movement to the patient.

The EMT-Basic then wraps the chest piece around the patient's chest and lifts the device as high as possible so that the side flaps rest in the patient's axilla. The EMT-Basic then applies the chest straps and tightens them. The EMT-Basic then applies the leg straps directly beneath the ischium and seesaws them into a vertical position crossing them over to the opposite side, attaching them and then tightening them.

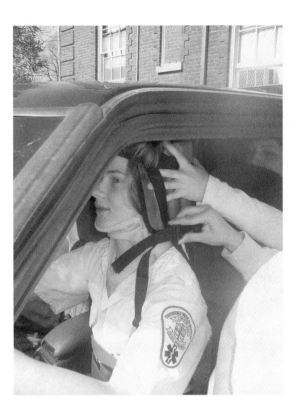

4. The patient's head is then secured into the top of the device so that the back of the device is touching the back of the patient's head.

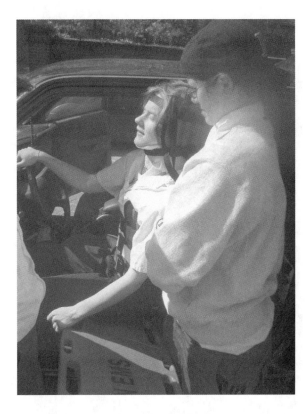

5. Retighten all straps. When the patient is lifted using KED straps, patient should not move.

APPLICATION OF A LONG SPINEBOARD

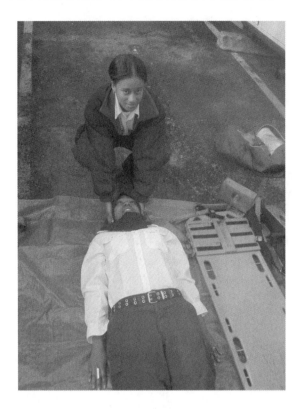

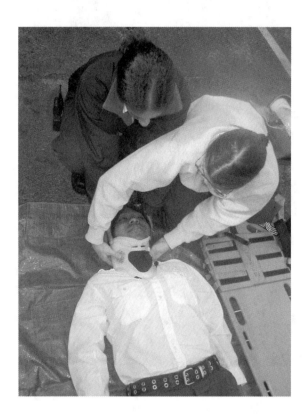

1. The EMT-Basic must first take manual stabilization of the cervical spine and indicate to the examiner that it is secure.

2. The EMT-Basic must then pass off stabilization to a partner without compromising constant stability and correctly size and apply a cervical collar.

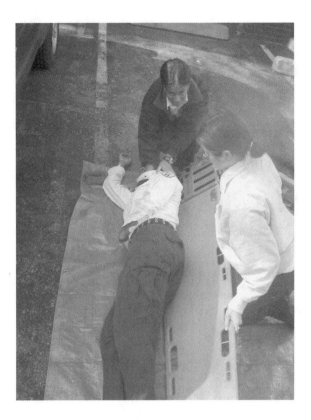

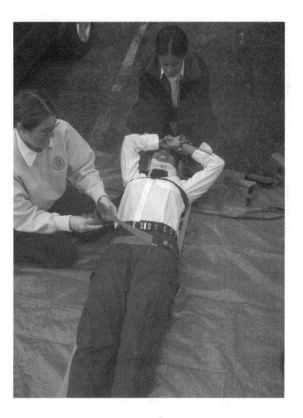

3. The EMT-Basic directs his or her crew of three, one holding the head and two at the patient's side to log roll the patient simultaneously at the command of the person holding the head. The EMT-Basic places the board beneath the patient and checks the back of the patient for injuries. Upon the EMT-Basic's direction, the person at the head commands the person to be rolled back to a supine position. The patient is positioned in the center of the board if necessary.

4. The patient is then secured to the board with a minimum of three straps: one across the chest, one across the pelvis, and one across the legs. No straps are to be placed on the abdomen and the buckles must be padded or placed where they do not touch the patient's body.

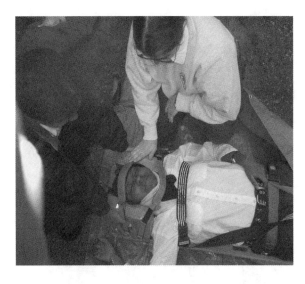

5. The head is then secured to the board with head blocks and straps.

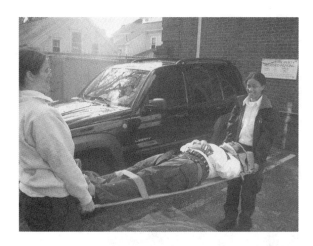

6. All straps are checked and retightened. When the board is turned on its side, the victim must not move. During this procedure at no time should any EMT-Basic step over the patient.

TRACTION SPLINTING

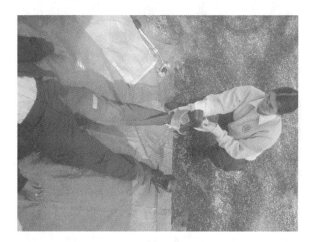

1. Assuming a mid-shaft closed femur fracture, the EMT-Basic indicates that he/she has checked for distal neural vital signs in both feet prior to application of traction. The EMT-Basic then positions the ankle strap/hitch on the ankle and takes manual traction, grasping the ring on the strap/hitch and supporting the lower leg. Traction is then passed to an assistant with no loss of traction.

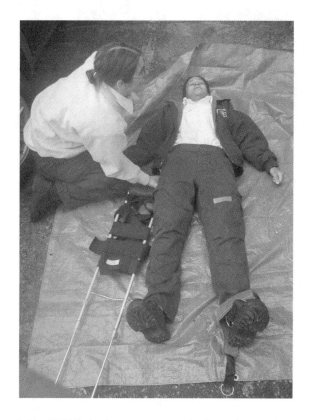

2. The EMT-Basic then prepares and adjusts the traction splint, using the uninjured leg as a guide. The EMT-Basic palpates the ischium and places the superior end of the splint adjacent to it and then lengthens it 8 to 12 inches beyond the end of the foot.

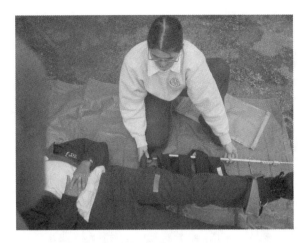

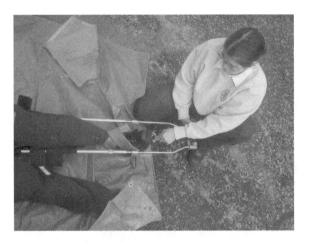

3. The EMT-Basic then places the splint next to the injured leg, palpates the ischium, and places the splint beneath the leg with the superior pad directly beneath the ischium. The ischium strap is then applied.

4. With the leg now lying on the splint, the traction winch is connected to the ankle strap/hitch and traction applied until the leg is tractioned to the same length as the uninjured leg, or until the patient indicates pain relief.

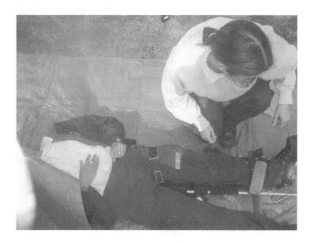

5. The leg straps are then applied, one below and above the site of the fracture superior to the knee and the other two on the lower leg.

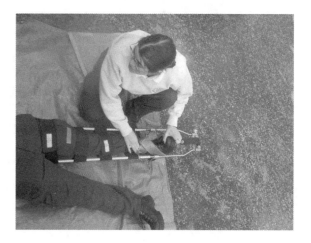

6. The EMT-Basic must indicate that he/she is again checking distal neural pulses and at no time must step over the patient.

Chapter Eight: **Pediatrics**

- Pediatric Populations

- Psychological and Social Factors

- Physical Differences

- Assessment

- Airway, Breathing, and Circulation

- Special Conditions

- Sudden Infant Death Syndrome (SIDS)

- Trauma

- Child Abuse and Neglect

- Special-Needs Infants and Children

- Family Response

The emergency medical care of infants and children is, like pediatrics itself, a very specific specialty. As one pediatrician likes to tell EMS-Basic students, infants and children are not just little adults. There are very real differences in pediatric anatomy and physiology, as well as psychology and sociological factors, which make the study of pediatrics in the prehospital setting a true specialty. In addition, the EMT-Basic must be prepared to deal with the caregivers of this group, who will present another dimension to the issue of providing quality care to the younger patient.

PEDIATRIC POPULATIONS

Some definitions of the subsets of the pediatric population are in order, since these subsets each present their own specific problems and concerns.

- **Neonates** are patients from the age of birth to 4 weeks.
- **Infants** are patients aged 4 weeks to 1 year.
- **Toddlers** are patients aged 1 to 3 years old.
- **Preschoolers** are patients aged 3 to 6 years old.
- **School-age children** are patients aged 6 to 12 years old.
- **Adolescents** are patients aged 12 to 18 years old.

Eighteen is usually considered the cutoff for pediatric care, although some special cases, such as chronic pediatric illnesses, may continue beyond the age of 18.

PSYCHOLOGICAL AND SOCIAL FACTORS

In performing assessment on a pediatric patient, the EMT-Basic must take into consideration psychological and sociological factors characteristic of this population. Toddlers and preschoolers generally will have a fear of separation from their parents or caregivers, and may be very suspicious of strangers. They may rebel at being touched or examined by strangers, and will be fearful of masks and needles. If one is available, a parent will best provide patient history, as the child may be unable to communicate important medical history and medication use.

School-age children and adolescents will be more social and open to EMT intervention, since they have usually begun social interaction in the school setting. Older adolescents may have to be assessed privately, since they might want to keep issues of sexual activity and substance abuse hidden from their parents.

PHYSICAL DIFFERENCES

The differences in airway anatomy present very real concerns to the EMT-Basic in treating these patients. Neonates and infants have larger tongues, smaller tracheas, and the epiglottis is located much higher in the airway. The EMT-Basic must also remember that neonates and infants cannot support their necks and heads, and that the EMT-Basic must always provide that support while holding or carrying the child. The heads of younger children are proportionally larger than those of older children and adults, which can present special problems in the case of trauma. In addition, vital signs of pediatric patients have different normal values from those of adults, with faster rates of heartbeat and respirations and lower average blood pressures.

ASSESSMENT

More so in pediatrics than in adult assessment, your initial overall impression of the patient's condition as you first observe the scene is most important. A child who is sick looks sick. When you approach the patient, you want to be as close to his or her emotional level as possible. Sick children have a very real fear of being sick, or even dying. Your presence must be reassuring and not threatening.

Assessment of mental status is accomplished by announcing your presence as you would with an adult and gauging the child's response to voice, touch, or painful stimuli. The EMT-Basic must ascertain whether the child's reaction to EMS presence is normal for a child of that age. It is a normal reaction, for example, for a toddler to cry as you approach, as a child this age will often cry at the approach of a uniformed stranger.

A big difference between adult and pediatric assessment is that the physical exam begins at the feet and works upward toward the head. Touching a child's head, especially among preschoolers, can increase anxiety levels, and it is better to have completed the rest of the body before this occurs.

When performing interventions and collecting vital signs, it is important that the devices used are properly sized for the size of the patient. The Bristow tape provides many of the sizes necessary for dealing with pediatric patients and is an important tool in pediatric assessment and treatment. An adult blood pressure cuff used on a pediatric patient will not give an accurate reading. It is also important to remember that "normal" vital signs are different for this group than for adults. Infants, for example, will have normal respiratory rates in the 40s, which would call for positive pressure ventilation support in the adult population.

Some common special concerns in the pediatric population include diseases that only occur in that age group, such as epiglottis and croup. Individual state protocols provide the assessment and interventions for these special conditions. One state, for example, allows for the administration of epinephrine via nebulae by EMT-Basics in the treatment of suspected croup or epiglottis with permission from medical control.

AIRWAY, BREATHING, AND CIRCULATION

Airway in the pediatric population should be quickly determined and the appropriate intervention taken if needed. Breathing is measured both for rate and quality, and circulation checked. It is important to begin oxygen therapy immediately for all children in respiratory distress and, in the event of severe respiratory distress, to provide for assistance in ventilation. The signs of severe respiratory distress are rates outside of the normal ranges, the presence of cyanosis, respiratory distress with poor muscle tone, and respiratory failure.

Pulses are checked on the brachial artery in the upper arm on smaller children. The absence of pulses is the indication to begin CPR, and the rate and method must be correct for the age of the child.

Airway

Neonates and infants are nose-breathers, so suctioning the nose with a bulb syringe can often clear up difficulty breathing in this group. In securing the airway of neonates and infants, the EMT-Basic must use care not to either hypoextend or hyperextend the neck and kink the very small airway. This can often be accomplished by placing a towel or blanket beneath the patient's shoulders, which will assist in keeping the head tilted at a more neutral position than would the full-head-chin lift technique that is used with adults. When inserting an oropharyngeal or nasopharyngeal airway, or when preparing to suction, the proper method of measuring the device is critical, and the properly sized device must be used. Inserting an oral airway in a pediatric patient is done only in the anatomical position, not rotated in, using a tongue depressor or laryngoscope blade to push the tongue out of the way.

Oxygen Therapy

As these patients will rarely accept a nasal cannula or pediatric face mask, oxygen therapy in neonates and infants can often be accomplished by using oxygen tubing and holding it two inches from the face of the patient. Simply flow the oxygen over the patient's nose and mouth, or hold a paper cup two inches away from the nose and mouth and blow the oxygen into the cup, creating an oxygen reservoir. In resuscitation, remember that the rates are faster and volume less, depending on the age and size of the patient.

SPECIAL CONDITIONS

Seizures

High core body temperatures resulting from infection usually cause pediatric seizures. These seizures are referred to as febrile seizures. A febrile seizure can be confirmed by checking the patient's forehead for a higher-than-normal temperature. If skin temperature is normal or below normal, then the cause of the seizure may be hypoxia, poisoning, trauma, hypoglycemia, or some other cause.

The patient's seizure history and medications should be determined. The patient's airway must be secured, the patient transported on his or her side, and oxygen therapy initiated. If the patient feels warm to the touch, a cool, damp towel applied to the head may be effective in lowering the body temperature enough to cancel the seizure. Remember that following a seizure, the patient will be postictal for a period of time.

Altered Mental Status

This condition may be caused by a variety of conditions, including seizures, hypoglycemia, poisoning, trauma, hypoxia, and shock. The treatment regimen is the same as with the adult population: secure the airway, administer oxygen, and transport.

Poisoning

Since children are curious, poisoning is a major cause of visits to the emergency room. If you suspect poisoning or overdose, you must make an effort while still on scene to locate the container that holds the substance ingested by the child, as this will give important information as to antidotes and treatment. If the patient is still responsive, contact medical control to check if ipecac or activated charcoal may be administered in accordance with local protocols. Ipecac is an emetic (causes vomiting) that will force the patient to expel the toxic substance. Ipecac is not given in cases of caustic poisoning or ingestion of petroleum products. Activated charcoal is an absorbent that will help prevent the toxin from being absorbed into the bloodstream. If the patient is unconscious, nothing may be given by mouth, as this may cause choking and an occluded airway. If unconscious, maintain the airway, administer oxygen, and transport priority.

Shock (Hypoperfusion)

In the pediatric population, unlike the adult population, shock is rarely a cardiac event, but is usually brought about by dehydration secondary to a variety of illnesses. Pediatric hypoperfusion is more problematic, since young children have a much lower blood supply than adults. It is important to note that low blood pressure in a pediatric patient is a late sign of hypoperfusion and requires a more aggressive approach to treatment than in an adult. In infants and toddlers, decreased urine output and dry crying (crying without tears) are good indicators of this condition.

Shocks in children calls for rapid transport with antishock measures as per the local protocols, including the use of an ALS intercept if indicated. These measures routinely include keeping the patient warm, elevating the legs, and administering of oxygen.

Near Drowning

It is important to remember, especially in pediatrics, that no one is dead until he or she is warm and dead. A cold, lifeless appearance of a near-drowning victim requires aggressive resuscitation efforts by EMS personnel and rapid transport to a pediatric trauma center. Good ventilation technique has resulted in the resuscitation of many children thought to be dead from near drowning in cold water. Respiratory distress is also a possibility with children who have suffered a near-drowning experience but were breathing fine after the event. Any victim of a near drowning should be transported to a pediatric emergency room for evaluation.

SUDDEN INFANT DEATH SYNDROME (SIDS)

There are few calls that are more traumatic in EMS than "child not breathing." SIDS is a condition in which a previously healthy infant is found his or her crib not breathing, and the post-mortem can find no cause for the death. It is important to remember that the patients in these calls include the parents of the child, and proper care means that someone must intervene with them, even if it requires calling for more personnel to the scene or a second rescue.

Many states require that resuscitative efforts be undertaken, even in the presence of biological death indicators such as rigor mortis and postmortem lividity, if for no other reason than to assure the parents that everything possible has been done for their child. While nothing will compensate for the loss of a child, a professional, assuring demeanor toward the parents may provide a small measure of comfort in this traumatic situation.

TRAUMA

Trauma, especially motor vehicle trauma, is the number-one cause of death in the pediatric population. Since the head is proportionally larger than the rest of a child's body, a head injury is more probable than in an adult. The bones of the body are more pliable and less likely to be fractured from blunt-force trauma. The pliability of the bones, however, means that the level of protection that they supply to the internal organs is less than in adults, and organ injuries are more common.

Assessment of trauma is as performed in adults, except that as in medical assessment, you should begin the physical exam at the feet and work toward the head in the case of a conscious patient. The treatment of pediatric trauma is essentially the same as for adult patients, although the use of PASG is dependent on local protocols and should not be used unless they fit properly.

CHILD ABUSE AND NEGLECT

It is a sad commentary on our society that child abuse and neglect are as prevalent as they are. EMS personnel are often the first to encounter these tragic victims. The definition of abuse is when improper or excessive action has caused harm or injury to someone. Abuse may be physical, psychological, or emotional in nature. Neglect is defined as insufficient attention or respect to someone with a claim to that attention. While these are somewhat subjective in nature, the EMT-Basic must always err on the side of the patient, and if there is any suspicion of abuse or neglect, it must be reported to the proper authorities. An infant left in a locked auto is an obvious case, but a ten-year-old left home alone is not quite as clear. Again, if there is any suspicion, the case must be reported to the proper authorities. Failure to report, in many jurisdictions, is a crime in itself, and can subject the EMT-Basic to criminal and civil penalties.

Multiple EMS interventions to the same address, or the same patient, also raise a flag of suspicion. Other signs and symptoms that there may be an abuse or neglect situation are unexplained bruises, injuries inconsistent with the explanation, conflicting stories of how the injury occurred, fresh burns, fear in the face of the child, and unconcern on the part of the parents.

An EMS intervention to a house where there is no adult present and small children are left alone may be a sign that the children are neglected. Other signs would include a child who appears malnourished, unsafe, or to be living in unhealthy living conditions, or with untreated chronic illnesses.

An infant who presents with possible central nervous system deficiencies may be suffering from shaken baby syndrome, in which violent shaking has damaged his or her spinal cord. This condition frequently leads to the death of the infant. The run report must be clear and concise as to the facts of the call in order to assist authorities in the proper disposition of this situation.

If the EMT-Basic suspects abuse or neglect, it is not his or her job to accuse the parents or caregivers. The EMT-Basic's proper concern is to care for the patient and to report any suspicions and facts uncovered to the proper authorities, usually the local police department. This information should also be presented to the receiving facility for proper treatment and follow-up by the hospital staff. In addition, some states require that this information be forwarded to the state agency responsible for children's health and safety. The EMT-Basic should report this directly and not merely rely on the police or hospital staff to do this. This is necessary, since this agency's interaction with the parent and patient may be the most crucial element in getting this child the proper care he or she deserves.

SPECIAL-NEEDS INFANTS AND CHILDREN

Many infants and children with chronic conditions are cared for at home by their parents and visiting health-care workers. If an emergency occurs, as it often does, a parent will call 911 for assistance, and EMS will respond and intervene. While EMT-Basic courses rarely go into detail on the emergency treatment of these conditions, the well-versed EMT tries to keep abreast of these procedures so that interventions are correct and in the best interest of the patient.

One of the most common conditions encountered by EMT-Basics is a tracheostomy tube that has been surgically implanted to the trachea of a child. These tubes may become plugged with mucus, which may cause the child to present with difficulty breathing. These tubes may be suctioned in the same manner as one would suction fluid from the oropharynx, remembering not to suction for more than five seconds and to administer oxygen to the tube between suctioning attempts. In the event of respiratory failure, the tube can be used to administer positive pressure ventilation directly to the trachea while blocking the nose and mouth. If a tube becomes dislodged or is removed by the patient, the stoma or opening can be used to ventilate and may have to be suctioned, especially if bleeding is present because of the removal of the tube. The EMT-Basic should not attempt to replace a tracheostomy tube that has been removed or dislodged, but should transport the child to the nearest pediatric care facility.

Children in chronic respiratory failure may be connected to a home ventilator. Parents are usually well instructed in the use of these devices, in addition to having backup systems in place. If EMS is called and none of these will operate properly, then the EMT-Basic must be prepared to manually ventilate the patient with an oxygen-supplied bag-valve mask and transport priority to the nearest facility.

Central lines are IV lines that have been placed in the larger veins of the torso in order to supply medication needed on a regular basis by the patient. Since IV lines are outside of the treatment protocols of an EMT-Basic, if complications from these lines are encountered, the patient must be transported to a pediatric hospital for proper management. EMT-Basic care should be to support the airway, assist respiration, and control any bleeding problems.

Gastrostomy tubes are tubes that are implanted directly into the stomach for children who cannot be fed by mouth. If these tubes become dislodged or plugged, and the parents have not been trained in their reinsertion, then the EMT-Basic must support breathing and transport the patient to the hospital for definitive care.

Shunts are tubes that are placed inside the skull to divert excess fluid to the stomach or to a reservoir on the side of the neck. If this device fails, the patient will present with signs of brain injury, such as change in mental status, seizures, nausea, vomiting, and loss of motor control. This patient has a severe condition and must be transported to the nearest facility with airway and respiratory support.

FAMILY RESPONSE

A child does not live alone, nor are infants, toddlers, and preschoolers capable of managing on their own. Any EMS calls involving this population, therefore, will present the EMT-Basic with multiple patients.

A child who is seriously injured or ill is almost always comforted by the presence of a parent or caregiver. (This may not be the case if the parent or caregiver is abusing the child.) The EMT-Basic is charged not only with caring for the child, but with reassuring the parents and assisting in lowering their anxiety. The general rule is that a calm parent will yield a calm child. The reverse is also true: an anxious parent will yield an anxious child, so it is prudent for the EMT-Basic to be conscious of the needs of the parent as well as the child.

In the event of a seriously ill or injured child, it is important to remember that the response of the parent may include anger or hysteria. The EMT-Basic must always choose whatever is best for his patient, the ill or injured child. This may be having the parent hold the child while both are properly secured to the ambulance stretcher, or it may require that the parent ride up front or even in another vehicle. If the parent is calm and can convey that calmness to the child, then allowing him or her to hold the child, or hold the oxygen mask, can go a long way to assist in calming the child.

Remember that the parents may have received specialized training for their child's medical care and they can be an important resource. Also remember that children are very perceptive and will quickly pick up on the EMT-Basic's confidence or uncertainty. It is important that the EMT-Basic project a well-trained and confident approach to the management of the pediatric patient.

PRACTICE SET

1. A pediatric patient who is 4 years old is categorized as a

   (A) Neonate

   (B) Infant

   (C) Toddler

   (D) Preschooler

2. An adolescent is defined as being in which age range?

   (A) 6 to 12 years old

   (B) 13 to 18 years old

   (C) 15 to 18 years old

   (D) 12 to 15 years old

3. The airway of an infant is proportionally _____ ___ the airway of an adolescent.

   (A) Smaller than

   (B) Larger than

   (C) The same size as

   (D) Inverse to

4. A six-month-old infant presents with difficulty breathing. Which characteristic of this child may account for this?

   (A) Proportionally larger head

   (B) Proportionally smaller trachea

   (C) Obligatory nose-breather

   (D) Higher respiratory rate

5. Which piece of equipment would be beneficial in treating the patient in question 4?

   (A) Nonrebreather mask

   (B) Vacuum suction unit

   (C) Bulb syringe

   (D) Magill forceps

6. Which sets of the vital signs listed below are considered normal for a neonate?

   (A) Pulse 140, respirations 40

   (B) Pulse 140, respirations 80

   (C) Pulse 80, respirations 40

   (D) Pulse 80, respirations 60

7. While performing the physical assessment on a three-year-old who fell off a wall and whose parents are not yet on scene, as you begin to palpate his neck, he begins to cry and tries to pull himself away from you. This action indicates which of the following?

   (A) Possible child abuse

   (B) Possible carotid-artery bruise

   (C) Possible pneumothorax

   (D) Possible cerebrovascular accident

8. Which of the following techniques should be used to open the airway of a one-year-old in respiratory arrest?

   (A) Head-tilt, chin-lift

   (B) Modified jaw thrust

   (C) Heimlich maneuver

   (D) Valsalva maneuver

9. Which of the following should NOT be used to administer oxygen to a pediatric patient?

   (A) Pediatric face mask

   (B) Paper cup and oxygen tubing

   (C) Blow-by technique

   (D) Oxygen-powered manual respirator

10. You should begin the physical examination of a pediatric patient at the

   (A) Head

   (B) Shoulders

   (C) Buttocks

   (D) Feet

11. The pulse that should be checked on an infant is located at the

    (A) Radial artery

    (B) Brachial artery

    (C) Carotid artery

    (D) Femoral artery

12. The most common cause of seizures in the pediatric population is

    (A) Poisoning

    (B) Hypoxia

    (C) Fever

    (D) Epilepsy

13. SIDS stands for

    (A) Sudden Idiopathic Dyspnea Syndrome

    (B) Surreptitious Insulin-Dependency Seizure

    (C) Sudden Infant Development Syndrome

    (D) Sudden Infant Death Syndrome

14. Which of the following need to be treated in a SIDS situation?

    (A) The infant

    (B) The parents

    (C) The EMS responders

    (D) All of the above

15. In examining a seven-year-old for a possible broken arm, you notice that his legs are covered with bruises. He cannot explain how they got there and appears withdrawn and defensive. You feel that this patient may be at risk for or a victim of child abuse. Which of the following should you immediately report this to?

    (A) The police

    (B) The receiving medical facility

    (C) The state agency charged with child protection

    (D) The media

ANSWER EXPLANATIONS

1. D

A four-year-old is a preschooler. Neonates are a day to 4 weeks old, infants 4 weeks to 1 year old, toddlers 1 to 3 years old.

2. B

You have to read this question and all of the answers carefully, since the correct range is defined as 12 to 18. Each answer contains partially correct ranges, but (B) is the most correct.

3. A

The infant's airway is proportionally smaller than that of the adolescent. Please note the presence of the key word *proportionally*.

4. C

Since neonates and infants are obligatory nose-breathers, the accumulation of mucus in the nasopharynx would cause dyspnea. The size of the head has nothing to do with breathing. A smaller trachea is problematic, but (C) is the better answer. Answer choice (D), while having to do with respirations, would not be directly related to causing dyspnea.

5. C

A bulb syringe is used to apply gentle suction and clear the nasal passages of mucus and will facilitate breathing. A nonrebreather mask is used for high-flow oxygen administration, a vacuum suction unit is too powerful to be used on a six-month-old, and Magill forceps are used to remove foreign bodies from the oropharynx and trachea.

6. A

Normal pulses for a newborn are in a range from 100 to 180. Respiratory rates are in a range of 30 to 60. If you were sure of the pulse range, you could eliminate the last two answers and focus on answer choices (A) or (B).

7. B

A carotid artery bruise would be painful to the touch and would increase the child's anxiety level. Child abuse is a tempting answer, except that the patient's response is fairly normal given the patient's age; he should be suspicious ofstrangers. There is nothing in the question that would indicate a pneumothorax or CVA.

8. B

The head-tilt-chin-lift may cause the airway of an infant to kink and obstruct, therefore the modified jaw thrust is the preferred method. The Heimlich maneuver is used to dislodge the airway obstruction of an adult, and, the Valsalva maneuver is taught to patients with supraventricular tachycardia.

9. D

(A), (B), and (C) are all methods of pediatric oxygen delivery. The manual oxygen-powered respirator should not be used in the pediatric population due to the risk of lung rupture from over-pressure.

10. D

Starting at the feet is the reverse of the physical examination technique for an adult. The reason for starting at the feet is that when you begin to examine the head, the anxiety level of the child will increase. If you have already examined the rest of the body, you will be in a good position to finish quickly and with a minimum of anxiety.

11. B

The brachial artery is the most accessible at this age.

12. C

While the other answer choices are all causes of seizures as well, most pediatric seizures are caused by high core temperatures.

13. D

Remember that it is important to read the question and all of the answers to determine the most correct one. Many people will answer (C) and not even read (D) simply because the first two words are part of the correct answer.

14. D

While your primary concern will be the infant in cardiopulmonary arrest, the parents will be anxious and concerned and need to be attended to as well. Since the question already states that this is a SIDS case, the outcome is not in question, and the EMS responders will need to be debriefed for Critical Incident Stress as well.

15. C

While it is advisable to notify the appropriate police department and the receiving medical facility of your suspicions, you are required in many states to notify the state agency responsible for child protection and this responsibility should not be left to other agencies but is the responsibility of the EMT Basic who has the suspicions. Obviously the media is not the appropriate agency to notify.

Chapter Nine: **Ambulance Operations**

- Preparation

- The Truck Check

- Dispatch

- En Route

- Arrival on Scene

- En Route to the Receiving Facility

- At the Receiving Facility

- Postrun

- Air Medical Considerations

All professional-grade EMT-Basics know that failure to plan is planning to fail. Every successful call depends on being physically and emotionally prepared to face the stresses of sudden illness, injury, hysteria, chaos, and even death. In addition, each on-duty EMT-Basic must be dressed in the uniform prescribed by the service. A professional appearance is vital if the EMT is to be taken seriously as a medical provider.

PREPARATION

Likewise, the equipment that an EMT-Basic must call upon to assist him or her must also be ready. It has happened that EMT-Basics have arrived on scene with empty oxygen bottles and dead batteries in their AEDs. This is not acceptable, and the performance of equipment can only be assured if its status and functionality are checked at the beginning of each shift. Likewise, street guides and maps, up-to-date protocols, and sufficient paperwork for the shift must also be verified as sufficient and ready.

A basic life-support EMS unit must have at least two licensed EMTs on board, one to drive and one to perform patient care. It is common procedure throughout a shift that the two EMTs rotate duties. In the event of a serious call, it is preferable for two licensed EMTs to be in the patient-care compartment, while a certified driver takes over the operation of the unit.

THE TRUCK CHECK

At the beginning of each shift, after being briefed by the personnel going off-duty as to the truck and the condition of supplies, the EMTs begin the ritual of the truck check. All operational details of the truck, such as fluid levels and functionality of all components, are verified and noted on the daily report. All medical supplies are inventoried and checked, and all pharmaceuticals are checked and expiration dates verified and noted. All equipment that uses portable batteries must be checked for sufficient voltage and working order, including pulse oximeters, glucometers, AED and cardiac monitors, and portable suction units. Depending on the service, each crew member may have a portable radio and/or a direct-connect cellular phone. The batteries on these devices should be changed to fresh batteries at the start of the shift and checked by contacting the dispatch center for a radio check. Also, at the beginning of each shift, the crew members should be clear as to their duties and responsibilities when a call is received, so that the execution of the call is as flawless as possible.

DISPATCH

When a call is received by the dispatcher, he or she notifies the responding unit by the means normally utilized by the service, either loudspeaker, radio, direct-connect cell phone, or in person if the dispatch center is in the same location as the unit. The dispatcher should relay to the responding EMS unit the location of the call, as well as the nature of the illness or injury and other special information that maybe useful to the responders. The dispatcher receiving the incoming call should also note the name of the caller and a callback number should more information be needed. This information is not normally broadcast to the responding unit.

EN ROUTE

When a call is received from the dispatcher, the crew chief acknowledges the call to the dispatcher. He or she repeats the location and nature of the call back to the dispatcher to assure that it is correctly received. If there is any confusion as to location or type of call, she should request clarification before acknowledging. The crew then responds quickly and enters their vehicle. All personnel secure themselves with the appropriate seat belts as the driver starts the engine. Before beginning to move, the driver checks to be sure that all doors are closed and that all personnel are ready.

Professional emergency vehicle drivers are physically and mentally fit at all times and alert of their surroundings and circumstances. They are intimately familiar with the vehicle they are driving, especially with its particular quirks. They anticipate the unexpected and avoid danger at all costs. They do not let the rush of adrenaline or excited radio traffic overcome their common sense and duty to drive safely. They are tolerant of the fact that others on the road may not be aware that they are responding to an emergency and may not yield the right of way, in spite of the EMS lights and sirens. While all states give specific privileges to emergency vehicles, these privileges do not permit the destruction of property or causing injury, and doing so will result in the appropriate penalties, as they would in the operation of any motor vehicle. It is always important to remember that the driver, not the senior EMT, is responsible for the operation of the vehicle, and is personally liable in the event of an accident.

Emergency lights and sirens should be used judiciously and as stated in particular state protocols. Extreme caution must always be used in approaching any intersection for cross traffic, regardless of the traffic control. Upon hearing a siren, some drivers will actually pull through a red stoplight into the path of an oncoming ambulance, thinking that the ambulance is behind them. Emergency vehicle operators must be aware that other emergency vehicles may be operating in priority mode and attempting to assert their right of way. It also should be noted that emergency vehicles never have the right of way over a stopped school bus with its red lights operating.

Police escorts are a dangerous practice and should only be utilized if the ambulance is unfamiliar with the location or the responding facility. Many times a police car attempting to escort an ambulance on a priority call will use its own lights and sirens to clear the roadway. However, vehicles that defer to the police car will often simply pull back into the path of the following ambulance after the police car has passed.

ARRIVAL ON SCENE

Once the unit is on scene, notify the dispatcher of this fact and give an update if the information you received was incorrect or incomplete. If the number of patients exceeds the capacity of the unit to handle, additional units must be requested at this time and MCI (mass casualty incident) procedures initiated.

The driver must position the vehicle safely and far enough away if the scene is hazardous or could become so. The crew chief should scan the scene for safety issues before committing the crew to a course of action. These include weapons, lack of police, electrical hazards, hazardous materials, and collapse dangers, among many others.

Once the scene is determined to be safe, the patient is approached and assessed. If there is a potential hazard, such as a vehicle on fire, then the patient must be moved before a proper assessment can be done. Whatever cervical spine stabilization can be done should be attempted, but should not hinder the prompt removal of the patient from the unsafe scene.

Once the patient is safely away from the hazard, then assessment is begun according to whether it is a trauma or medical scenario, and proper treatments initiated. Once the patient is properly triaged and treated, he is ready for transport, unless this was earlier determined to be a load-and-go injury and you are already en route.

EN ROUTE TO THE RECEIVING FACILITY

Once en route to the receiving facility, the driver notifies dispatch of that fact, and the EMT-Basic responsible for treating the patient collects the information necessary to notify the receiving facility. It is important to paint as clear a picture as possible so that the receiving facility knows the condition of the patient en route and can prepare accordingly. The facility should be informed of the patient's chief complaint, pertinent findings from the assessments, vital signs, and estimated time of arrival.

While en route, it is also important to remember the patient's emotional state if he or she is conscious. It is part of good patient care to assure your patient that he or she is in the care of a competent provider and receiving optimal care. A patient will quickly sense if the EMT-Basic is unsure of herself, and become anxious. In addition, vital signs should continue to be monitored according to local protocols in order to monitor any changes in the patient's condition.

AT THE RECEIVING FACILITY

Once at the receiving facility, the driver notifies dispatch of this fact and goes to the rear of the vehicle to assist in removing the patient. The patient is brought to the triage area and transferred to hospital care by the direction of the receiving nurse or physician. A complete oral report is given to the initial hospital caregiver along with a copy of the written report containing the pertinent information from the assessments, vital signs, and EMT interventions.

POSTRUN

Once back at the station, the truck should be restocked. The run report should be completed after obtaining the times from the dispatcher and filed in a locked bin according to local protocols regarding confidentiality of patient-care information. Disposable supplies are restocked and clean linens used to make up the stretcher. Once everything has been cleaned, disinfected, and restocked, the unit is available for another run. Dispatch is notified that the unit is back in service.

AIR MEDICAL CONSIDERATIONS

Local protocols will often dictate when air transport is indicated and how it is to be used. One state, for example, requires any patient with a trauma score less than 11 and more than 20 minutes from the trauma center be sent by air if appropriate.

Unfortunately, many other factors come into play in this type of scenario besides land transport time and trauma score. Helicopters will not fly, for example, in snow and ice storms, when EMS calls are frequent and often serious. Too often precious time is lost by a crew chief ordering a helicopter and preparing a patient for helicopter transfer, and then finding out that the helicopter is not available.

The crew chief must make his or her decision based upon all of these considerations. In addition, he or she must establish a landing zone for the helicopter. A landing zone must be at least 100 by 100 feet, fairly level, paved or grass-covered if possible, and free from overhead obstructions, particularly electrical wires. The landing zone should have a fire truck in attendance, as well as emergency lighting if at night and unlit. Areas using helicopters are well advised to establish designated helicopter landing zones and to have live practices at these sites. This will help prevent problems when trying to accomplish a helicopter transfer of a critical patient under marginal conditions.

No one should approach the helicopter until instructed to do so by the pilot or a helicopter crew member. Helicopters will not routinely shut down for a patient transfer due to the amount of time it takes to power down and back up again, so the blades are often rotating while the patient is being transferred. The helicopter crews are the experts in this type of operation, and their instructions should be followed completely. As a general rule, always approach a helicopter from the front or side in view of the pilot, keeping your head down. Never approach from the rear. If the helicopter is on a slight slope, be aware that the clearance of the main rotors will be dangerously low on the uphill side and may be unapproachable there.

PRACTICE SET

1. Ambulances should be supplied with

   (A) Only those supplies that the service can afford.

   (B) All of the supplies necessary for the operations for which the ambulance is licensed.

   (C) An emergency childbirth kit.

   (D) Safety equipment mandated by the licensing authority.

2. A person providing treatment to an injured person in the patient compartment of an ambulance must be

   (A) A First Responder

   (B) A licensed EMT

   (C) A licensed registered nurse

   (D) Over four feet tall

3. As you begin your shift, you receive a priority dispatch for a patient in respiratory distress at a local nursing home. You have not yet performed the mandatory truck check. What should you do?

   (A) Disregard the check and let the next shift do it.

   (B) Do not respond to any calls until the check is completed.

   (C) Respond to the call and perform the check when you return in service.

   (D) Have the driver perform the check while the EMT assesses the patient.

4. Which of the following does not rely on an electrical battery?

   (A) Pulse oximeter

   (B) Portable oxygen tank

   (C) Glucometer

   (D) Portable suction unit

5. Your EMS radio announces, "Rescue 1, respond to 123 Main Street for a man fallen off a ladder with head laceration, possibly unconscious, time out 15:30 hours." Your response to dispatch should be

   (A) "10-4."

   (B) "Roger."

   (C) "Rescue 1 responding priority to 123 Main Street for a male possibly unconscious with a head laceration."

   (D) "Rescue 1 responding with two EMTs, Basic Life Support only, lights and sirens, to 123 Main Street in Anytown for a male who has fallen off of a ladder and has a possible skull fracture. We are responding at 15:31 hours. Do you copy, dispatch?"

6. While responding priority to a hospital with a critical patient upon whom CPR is being performed, you approach a school bus that has stopped to discharge students and has its red lights flashing. The correct course of action is to

   (A) Disregard the school bus and pass it on the left using lights and sirens.

   (B) Stop behind the bus and wait until the driver shuts off his flashing lights and signals you to pass.

   (C) Pull alongside the bus while continuing to operate your lights and sirens so that the school bus driver knows you are responding priority.

   (D) Request police escort to pass the bus.

7. You respond priority to a motor vehicle accident. Arriving on scene, you notice a car has struck a fuel, tank truck broadside and liquid is running downhill toward you. The best place to park your ambulance is

   (A) At the spot you first noticed the liquid.

   (B) Past the vehicle, uphill from the liquid spill.

   (C) Directly next to the vehicle to expedite patient care and transfer.

   (D) 250 feet from the crash.

8. You should notify the receiving facility of a critically ill patient

   (A) At the time of dispatch.

   (B) En route to the hospital.

   (C) Never.

   (D) At the conclusion of the rapid assessment.

ANSWER EXPLANATIONS

1. B

The minimum list of supplies is usually mandated by the licensing authority, but the service should be carrying everything necessary for the operations for which the ambulance is licensed, whether Basic Life Support, Advanced Life Support, Pediatric Transport, Neonate Transport, etc. Answer choices (C) and (D) are partially correct since any BLS ambulance should have them, but answer (B) is the best answer.

2. B

First responders are public safety personnel who may be on the scene with an injured or ill person, but once a licensed EMS vehicle is on scene, care is transferred to the licensed EMT-Basic who arrives with the vehicle. Registered nurses routinely work in the hospital setting, and nursing licensure is not a requirement to provide prehospital care; however, licensure as an EMT-Basic is. Height has no relation to this question.

3. C

The check should be performed by each shift and not be relegated to the next shift. Patient care is always a priority, so it would be inappropriate to neglect the response to a priority call. A call for respiratory distress is going to require both crew persons, so answer choice (D) is incorrect as well.

4. B

The portable oxygen tank does not rely on an electric battery. (A) and (C) are definitely battery operated. (D) is questionable, since portable suction units can be either electrically or manually operated. Again, all answers must be read and the best answer chosen.

5. C

If the information was not heard properly, it is possible that the unit could respond to the wrong location, so repeating the dispatch information is always prudent. (A) and (B) are merely acknowledgments. (D) is too long, relays back information that is not pertinent, and attempts a diagnosis without even seeing the patient. This ties up the radio frequency unnecessarily.

6. B

A school bus has the right of way over emergency vehicles in all situations. Answer choices (A) and (C) are moving violations and will subject the ambulance driver to criminal and civil sanctions. Answer choice (D) is incorrect since a police car has the same rules of operation as an ambulance and can't pass the school bus either.

7. B

The uphill parking place will put your vehicle out of the path of this potentially dangerous spill. (A) is incorrect because the liquid is continuing to spill and will soon be underneath your vehicle, putting it directly in a hazardous situation. Answer choice (C) is incorrect since parking that close to a leaking fuel truck is dangerous to the vehicle, crew, and patient. (D) is incomplete and should be discarded.

8. B

En route to the receiving facility is the correct answer. Answer choice (A) is incorrect, since at this point you do not have enough information for the receiving facility to begin their preparations for this patient. Answer choice (C) is incorrect, since you always want to notify them so that they can be ready. Answer choice (D) is also incorrect, since you still do not have all of the information needed.

Full-Length Practice Test and Explanations

Practice Test
Answer Sheet

Remove (or photocopy) this answer sheet and use it to complete the practice test. See the answer key following the test when finished. For an analysis of your score, see "Your Practice Test Score," following the practice test answers and explanations section.

1. Ⓐ Ⓑ Ⓒ Ⓓ	31. Ⓐ Ⓑ Ⓒ Ⓓ	61. Ⓐ Ⓑ Ⓒ Ⓓ	91. Ⓐ Ⓑ Ⓒ Ⓓ	121. Ⓐ Ⓑ Ⓒ Ⓓ
2. Ⓐ Ⓑ Ⓒ Ⓓ	32. Ⓐ Ⓑ Ⓒ Ⓓ	62. Ⓐ Ⓑ Ⓒ Ⓓ	92. Ⓐ Ⓑ Ⓒ Ⓓ	122. Ⓐ Ⓑ Ⓒ Ⓓ
3. Ⓐ Ⓑ Ⓒ Ⓓ	33. Ⓐ Ⓑ Ⓒ Ⓓ	63. Ⓐ Ⓑ Ⓒ Ⓓ	93. Ⓐ Ⓑ Ⓒ Ⓓ	123. Ⓐ Ⓑ Ⓒ Ⓓ
4. Ⓐ Ⓑ Ⓒ Ⓓ	34. Ⓐ Ⓑ Ⓒ Ⓓ	64. Ⓐ Ⓑ Ⓒ Ⓓ	94. Ⓐ Ⓑ Ⓒ Ⓓ	124. Ⓐ Ⓑ Ⓒ Ⓓ
5. Ⓐ Ⓑ Ⓒ Ⓓ	35. Ⓐ Ⓑ Ⓒ Ⓓ	65. Ⓐ Ⓑ Ⓒ Ⓓ	95. Ⓐ Ⓑ Ⓒ Ⓓ	125. Ⓐ Ⓑ Ⓒ Ⓓ
6. Ⓐ Ⓑ Ⓒ Ⓓ	36. Ⓐ Ⓑ Ⓒ Ⓓ	66. Ⓐ Ⓑ Ⓒ Ⓓ	96. Ⓐ Ⓑ Ⓒ Ⓓ	126. Ⓐ Ⓑ Ⓒ Ⓓ
7. Ⓐ Ⓑ Ⓒ Ⓓ	37. Ⓐ Ⓑ Ⓒ Ⓓ	67. Ⓐ Ⓑ Ⓒ Ⓓ	97. Ⓐ Ⓑ Ⓒ Ⓓ	127. Ⓐ Ⓑ Ⓒ Ⓓ
8. Ⓐ Ⓑ Ⓒ Ⓓ	38. Ⓐ Ⓑ Ⓒ Ⓓ	68. Ⓐ Ⓑ Ⓒ Ⓓ	98. Ⓐ Ⓑ Ⓒ Ⓓ	128. Ⓐ Ⓑ Ⓒ Ⓓ
9. Ⓐ Ⓑ Ⓒ Ⓓ	39. Ⓐ Ⓑ Ⓒ Ⓓ	69. Ⓐ Ⓑ Ⓒ Ⓓ	99. Ⓐ Ⓑ Ⓒ Ⓓ	129. Ⓐ Ⓑ Ⓒ Ⓓ
10. Ⓐ Ⓑ Ⓒ Ⓓ	40. Ⓐ Ⓑ Ⓒ Ⓓ	70. Ⓐ Ⓑ Ⓒ Ⓓ	100. Ⓐ Ⓑ Ⓒ Ⓓ	130. Ⓐ Ⓑ Ⓒ Ⓓ
11. Ⓐ Ⓑ Ⓒ Ⓓ	41. Ⓐ Ⓑ Ⓒ Ⓓ	71. Ⓐ Ⓑ Ⓒ Ⓓ	101. Ⓐ Ⓑ Ⓒ Ⓓ	131. Ⓐ Ⓑ Ⓒ Ⓓ
12. Ⓐ Ⓑ Ⓒ Ⓓ	42. Ⓐ Ⓑ Ⓒ Ⓓ	72. Ⓐ Ⓑ Ⓒ Ⓓ	102. Ⓐ Ⓑ Ⓒ Ⓓ	132. Ⓐ Ⓑ Ⓒ Ⓓ
13. Ⓐ Ⓑ Ⓒ Ⓓ	43. Ⓐ Ⓑ Ⓒ Ⓓ	73. Ⓐ Ⓑ Ⓒ Ⓓ	103. Ⓐ Ⓑ Ⓒ Ⓓ	133. Ⓐ Ⓑ Ⓒ Ⓓ
14. Ⓐ Ⓑ Ⓒ Ⓓ	44. Ⓐ Ⓑ Ⓒ Ⓓ	74. Ⓐ Ⓑ Ⓒ Ⓓ	104. Ⓐ Ⓑ Ⓒ Ⓓ	134. Ⓐ Ⓑ Ⓒ Ⓓ
15. Ⓐ Ⓑ Ⓒ Ⓓ	45. Ⓐ Ⓑ Ⓒ Ⓓ	75. Ⓐ Ⓑ Ⓒ Ⓓ	105. Ⓐ Ⓑ Ⓒ Ⓓ	135. Ⓐ Ⓑ Ⓒ Ⓓ
16. Ⓐ Ⓑ Ⓒ Ⓓ	46. Ⓐ Ⓑ Ⓒ Ⓓ	76. Ⓐ Ⓑ Ⓒ Ⓓ	106. Ⓐ Ⓑ Ⓒ Ⓓ	136. Ⓐ Ⓑ Ⓒ Ⓓ
17. Ⓐ Ⓑ Ⓒ Ⓓ	47. Ⓐ Ⓑ Ⓒ Ⓓ	77. Ⓐ Ⓑ Ⓒ Ⓓ	107. Ⓐ Ⓑ Ⓒ Ⓓ	137. Ⓐ Ⓑ Ⓒ Ⓓ
18. Ⓐ Ⓑ Ⓒ Ⓓ	48. Ⓐ Ⓑ Ⓒ Ⓓ	78. Ⓐ Ⓑ Ⓒ Ⓓ	108. Ⓐ Ⓑ Ⓒ Ⓓ	138. Ⓐ Ⓑ Ⓒ Ⓓ
19. Ⓐ Ⓑ Ⓒ Ⓓ	49. Ⓐ Ⓑ Ⓒ Ⓓ	79. Ⓐ Ⓑ Ⓒ Ⓓ	109. Ⓐ Ⓑ Ⓒ Ⓓ	139. Ⓐ Ⓑ Ⓒ Ⓓ
20. Ⓐ Ⓑ Ⓒ Ⓓ	50. Ⓐ Ⓑ Ⓒ Ⓓ	80. Ⓐ Ⓑ Ⓒ Ⓓ	110. Ⓐ Ⓑ Ⓒ Ⓓ	140. Ⓐ Ⓑ Ⓒ Ⓓ
21. Ⓐ Ⓑ Ⓒ Ⓓ	51. Ⓐ Ⓑ Ⓒ Ⓓ	81. Ⓐ Ⓑ Ⓒ Ⓓ	111. Ⓐ Ⓑ Ⓒ Ⓓ	141. Ⓐ Ⓑ Ⓒ Ⓓ
22. Ⓐ Ⓑ Ⓒ Ⓓ	52. Ⓐ Ⓑ Ⓒ Ⓓ	82. Ⓐ Ⓑ Ⓒ Ⓓ	112. Ⓐ Ⓑ Ⓒ Ⓓ	142. Ⓐ Ⓑ Ⓒ Ⓓ
23. Ⓐ Ⓑ Ⓒ Ⓓ	53. Ⓐ Ⓑ Ⓒ Ⓓ	83. Ⓐ Ⓑ Ⓒ Ⓓ	113. Ⓐ Ⓑ Ⓒ Ⓓ	143. Ⓐ Ⓑ Ⓒ Ⓓ
24. Ⓐ Ⓑ Ⓒ Ⓓ	54. Ⓐ Ⓑ Ⓒ Ⓓ	84. Ⓐ Ⓑ Ⓒ Ⓓ	114. Ⓐ Ⓑ Ⓒ Ⓓ	144. Ⓐ Ⓑ Ⓒ Ⓓ
25. Ⓐ Ⓑ Ⓒ Ⓓ	55. Ⓐ Ⓑ Ⓒ Ⓓ	85. Ⓐ Ⓑ Ⓒ Ⓓ	115. Ⓐ Ⓑ Ⓒ Ⓓ	145. Ⓐ Ⓑ Ⓒ Ⓓ
26. Ⓐ Ⓑ Ⓒ Ⓓ	56. Ⓐ Ⓑ Ⓒ Ⓓ	86. Ⓐ Ⓑ Ⓒ Ⓓ	116. Ⓐ Ⓑ Ⓒ Ⓓ	146. Ⓐ Ⓑ Ⓒ Ⓓ
27. Ⓐ Ⓑ Ⓒ Ⓓ	57. Ⓐ Ⓑ Ⓒ Ⓓ	87. Ⓐ Ⓑ Ⓒ Ⓓ	117. Ⓐ Ⓑ Ⓒ Ⓓ	147. Ⓐ Ⓑ Ⓒ Ⓓ
28. Ⓐ Ⓑ Ⓒ Ⓓ	58. Ⓐ Ⓑ Ⓒ Ⓓ	88. Ⓐ Ⓑ Ⓒ Ⓓ	118. Ⓐ Ⓑ Ⓒ Ⓓ	148. Ⓐ Ⓑ Ⓒ Ⓓ
29. Ⓐ Ⓑ Ⓒ Ⓓ	59. Ⓐ Ⓑ Ⓒ Ⓓ	89. Ⓐ Ⓑ Ⓒ Ⓓ	119. Ⓐ Ⓑ Ⓒ Ⓓ	149. Ⓐ Ⓑ Ⓒ Ⓓ
30. Ⓐ Ⓑ Ⓒ Ⓓ	60. Ⓐ Ⓑ Ⓒ Ⓓ	90. Ⓐ Ⓑ Ⓒ Ⓓ	120. Ⓐ Ⓑ Ⓒ Ⓓ	150. Ⓐ Ⓑ Ⓒ Ⓓ

Practice Test

1. Which of the following is an example of an unsafe scene for an EMT to enter?

   (A) Fifty-four-year-old male with difficulty breathing

   (B) Twenty-three-year-old female with abdominal pain

   (C) Eighteen-year-old adolescent with a gunshot wound to the chest

   (D) Four-year-old child with leg pain

2. The arterioles connect the _____ and the capillaries.

   (A) Veins

   (B) Venules

   (C) Arteries

   (D) Vena cavae

3. Which of the following patients is at greatest risk for hypothermia?

   (A) Thirty-year-old firefighter

   (B) Twelve-year-old skier

   (C) Forty-five-year-old EMT

   (D) Seventy-year-old librarian

4. Which of the following is not one of the five stages of grief?

   (A) Denial

   (B) Anger

   (C) Crying

   (D) Acceptance

5. The zygomatic bones are located in the

   (A) Chest

   (B) Lower leg

   (C) Back

   (D) Face

6. Which of the following patients is competent to give expressed consent?

   (A) Five-year-old patient with a leg fracture

   (B) Intoxicated male, unconscious and unresponsive to any stimuli

   (C) Mentally challenged patient in a group home

   (D) Eighteen-year-old female with abdominal pain

7. When using air transport, the EMT should approach a helicopter

   (A) From the uphill side.

   (B) From the rear.

   (C) Only when instructed by a helicopter crew member.

   (D) Under no circumstances, but instead allow the crew to come to them.

8. Which of the following should be noted as insignificant in conducting the patient assessment?

   (A) Medication bottles

   (B) Comments of bystanders and family members

   (C) Physical condition of the patient

   (D) Patient's medical insurance

KAPLAN

9. Which of the following is not a component of the Glasgow Coma Scale?

   (A) Eye opening
   (B) Verbal response
   (C) Motor response
   (D) Tactile sensatory response

10. In which of the following situations is it NOT necessary to notify law enforcement or health department officials?

    (A) Child abuse
    (B) Sexually transmitted diseases
    (C) A person about to commit a criminal act
    (D) Patient with a history of treatment for AIDS

11. The head is _____ to the chest.

    (A) Inferior
    (B) Anterior
    (C) Superior
    (D) Posterior

12. Which of the following parts of the body are NOT checked for DCAP-BTLS in the focused trauma assessment?

    (A) Head
    (B) Torso
    (C) Extremities
    (D) Genitals

13. There are _____ vertebrae in the lumbar section.

    (A) 5
    (B) 12
    (C) 14
    (D) 19

14. Signs and symptoms of post-traumatic stress disorder include the following except

    (A) Loss of sexual desire
    (B) Loss of appetite
    (C) Loss of interest in work
    (D) Loss of spontaneity

15. The letter "G" in the APGAR score stands for

    (A) Grating
    (B) Grimace
    (C) Guarding
    (D) Gurgling

16. You are dispatched to an auto accident on a local city street. You respond priority and arrive on scene with suitable precautions. The police are on scene. There is one victim, a woman seated in the car. Her car backed into another car as she was pulling out of her driveway at low speed. As you approach the car, she advises you that she is 36 weeks pregnant with her first child. She advises you that she has no injuries and no hemorrhaging, and is not in any pain; however, she wishes to be checked out at the hospital. In what position should she be transported?

    (A) Trendelenburg
    (B) Fowler
    (C) Left lateral recumbent
    (D) Right lateral recumbent

17. Which of the following is NOT a significant risk factor for suicide?

    (A) Male over 40 years of age
    (B) History of alcohol or drug abuse
    (C) Previous history of suicide attempts
    (D) Bankruptcy

18. You respond to a call for a female acting strangely. You respond nonpriority and are met by the police, who request you transport the patient to a hospital for a psychological evaluation. The patient is a twenty-year-old female who is ballet dancing in the supermarket, bowing and throwing kisses to an imaginary audience. When you approach her, she smiles at you and introduces you to her imaginary dancing partner, Rudolf Nureyev. You should next

    (A) Pretend to shake Mr. Nureyev's hand.
    (B) Wrap your arms around the patient and force her to the stretcher.
    (C) Gently explain to her that there is no Mr. Nureyev dancing with her.
    (D) Tackle the patient and assist the police in handcuffing her hands behind her back.

19. A neonate will normally have _____ pulse rates and respiratory rates than an infant.

    (A) Higher
    (B) Lower
    (C) More irregular
    (D) Less irregular

20. Most EMTs are injured at which of the following types of calls?

    (A) Domestic violence calls
    (B) Motor vehicle accidents
    (C) Workplace injury calls
    (D) In-station accidents

21. Veins are blood vessels that carry deoxygenated blood _____ the heart.

    (A) Into
    (B) Away from
    (C) Toward
    (D) From the lungs to

22. Which of the following is not a type of muscle?

    (A) Voluntary
    (B) Involuntary
    (C) Cardiac
    (D) Regulatory

23. Which of the following is not a component of the SAMPLE survey?

    (A) Signs and symptoms
    (B) Allergies
    (C) Medications
    (D) Pulse rate

24. When should EMS communication equipment be checked?

    (A) Daily
    (B) Monthly
    (C) Weekly
    (D) At the start of every shift

25. The first thing to be considered when arriving on scene of an emergency call is

    (A) Scene safety
    (B) Universal precautions
    (C) Airway
    (D) Breathing

26. What is the legal degree of intoxication for a person to be judged incompetent to refuse medical care?

    (A) .08 percent
    (B) .1 percent
    (C) 1 percent
    (D) There is no legal limit

27. Once you have determined that the scene is safe and you are wearing the proper universal precautions, the next thing to be checked is

(A) Airway
(B) Breathing
(C) Circulation
(D) Gross hemorrhage

28. Which of the following is not a level of consciousness?

(A) Alert
(B) Conscious
(C) Active
(D) Oriented

29. Perfusion in patient assessment refers to

(A) Amount of fluid in the lungs.
(B) Amount of oxygen in the hemoglobin.
(C) Amount of urine in the bladder.
(D) Amount of blood in the heart.

30. Hypothermic is best described as

(A) Too hot
(B) Too cold
(C) Too sweaty
(D) Too dry

31. You are dispatched to a residence for a man down. You respond priority and arrive on scene wearing suitable precautions. The scene is safe. You enter the bedroom, and the patient's wife advises you that he is being treated for lung cancer and is undergoing chemotherapy. The patient presents on the primary assessment as unresponsive with no gag reflex. His airway is open, he is breathing spontaneously at a rate of 12, and he has a weak thready pulse rate of 100. You insert an oropharyngeal airway and administer supplemental oxygen via a nonrebreather mask at a flow rate of 12 lpm. Your transport time to the nearest hospital emergency room is 30 minutes, but there is an ALS unit 15 minutes out. You should next

(A) Call for an ALS intercept.
(B) Begin priority transport.
(C) Administer .3mg epinephrine subcutaneously.
(D) Request an air transport.

32. The letter "Q" in the acronym OPQRST stands for

(A) Quantity
(B) Quality
(C) Quasi
(D) Quick

33. After the focused trauma assessment is completed on a trauma patient, the assessment should be rechecked every:

(A) Two minutes
(B) Five minutes
(C) Ten minutes
(D) Fifteen minutes

34. Which of the following trauma calls is a "load and go"?

(A) Fall from a fourth-story window
(B) Motor vehicle accident at an intersection
(C) Open femur fracture
(D) Adult bicycle accident

35. In the mnemonic DCAP-BTLS, the letter "B" stands for

    (A) Bruising
    (B) Brittleness
    (C) Burns
    (D) Bradycardia

36. A patient viewed from the side is bisected by the

    (A) Midaxillary line
    (B) Midclavicular line
    (C) Midsternal line
    (D) Horizontal plane

37. You are dispatched to a man who has fallen from a garage roof. You respond priority and arrive on scene wearing suitable precautions. The scene is safe. The patient is a thirty-two-year-old male who is conscious, but confused as to events. You are holding stabilization while your partner completes the focused trauma assessment. Which device should be applied following the focused assessment of the head and neck?

    (A) Halo traction device
    (B) Hare traction device
    (C) Hale splint
    (D) Cervical collar

38. The Good Samaritan Act is

    (A) A religious doctrine.
    (B) A statute that minimizes liability for certain acts.
    (C) A good deed done by an EMT.
    (D) A play put on by EMTs to entertain children.

39. While en route to the hospital with a critically ill patient, how often should you repeat vital signs as part of ongoing assessment?

    (A) Every one minute
    (B) Every three minutes
    (C) Every five minutes
    (D) Every ten minutes

40. The "U" in the mnemonic AVPU means

    (A) Uniform
    (B) Unequivocal
    (C) Unknown
    (D) Unconscious

41. Which of the following should never be given over the two-way radio system?

    (A) The location of a call
    (B) The nature of a call
    (C) The patient's name
    (D) The EMT's name

42. Which of the following is not a required part of a prehospital care report?

    (A) Patient's name
    (B) Patient's date of birth
    (C) Patient's gender
    (D) Patient's medical insurance information

43. You are dispatched to the local high school for an eye injury. You respond priority and arrive on scene, the scene is safe, and you are wearing suitable precautions. You are directed to the nurse's office, where you find a sixteen-year-old male with a pencil stuck in his left eye. All vital signs are normal, and there is no other injury. You should dress and bandage

    (A) His left eye.
    (B) Both eyes.
    (C) His entire upper head.
    (D) A dressing is not indicated.

44. Which of the following situations must be reported by EMTs if they become aware of them?

    (A) Child abuse
    (B) Sexual abuse
    (C) Elderly abuse
    (D) Spousal abuse

45. When is the umbilical cord cut?

    (A) Immediately after the baby is delivered

    (B) When it ceases pulsing

    (C) When the placenta is delivered

    (D) At the hospital

46. Which of the following is not a sign or symptom of hypovolemic shock?

    (A) Dropping blood pressure

    (B) Excessive thirst

    (C) Tachypnea

    (D) Bradycardia

47. A competent patient may refuse which of the following procedures?

    (A) Cervical stabilization with a cervical collar

    (B) Spinal immobilization with a spine board

    (C) Intravenous fluid administration

    (D) Any medical procedure

48. Oxygen is normally administered to a patient

    (A) By Injection

    (B) By Inhalation

    (C) Orally

    (D) Sublingually

49. SIDS normally occurs between the ages of

    (A) 0 and 1

    (B) 1 and 2

    (C) 2 and 3

    (D) 3 and 4

50. An impaled object should never be removed unless

    (A) Ordered to do so by police on scene.

    (B) Requested by patient.

    (C) It interferes with airway management.

    (D) It is longer than 12 inches.

51. An EMT-Basic must check which of the following when administering pharmaceuticals?

    (A) Color of drug

    (B) Contraindications

    (C) Side effects

    (D) Expiration date

52. Which of the following patient positions indicates serious respiratory difficulty?

    (A) Semi-Fowler position

    (B) Hundrek's position

    (C) Tripod position

    (D) Supine position

53. The contraction of the ventricles produces the _____ pressure in the arteries.

    (A) Systolic

    (B) Diastolic

    (C) Arterial

    (D) Static

54. On a cold winter day, you respond to a local pond for an ice fisherman who fell through the ice. You arrive on scene and you observe a male lying supine in cold and wet clothes; the patient has no pulse or respirations. A scuba diver advises that your patient has been underwater for the 30 minutes it took the diver to suit up and effect the rescue. You should next

    (A) Pronounce the patient dead.

    (B) Immediately begin CPR.

    (C) Place the patient in the truck, remove his wet clothes and begin to warm him.

    (D) Reequest an ALS intercept.

55. You are dispatched to a local health club for a male with difficulty breathing. You respond priority and arrive on scene. The scene is safe and you are wearing suitable precautions. You observe a 30-year-old male patient with obvious dyspnea, pale, and mildly diaphoretic. He has a history of asthma, blood pressure of 150/80, pulse of 110, and respiratory rate of 24. His pulse oximetry saturation is 88 percent on room air. Which of the following oxygen delivery devices should you apply?

(A) Nasal cannula

(B) Simple face mask

(C) Partial non-rebreather

(D) Full non-rebreather

56. In the scenario in question 55, what flow rate will you set your oxygen regulator to?

(A) 4 liters per minute

(B) 10 liters per minute

(C) 15 liters per minute

(D) 20 liters per minute

57. Which of the following is not a landmark for a lung field you would auscultate in question 55?

(A) Anterior midclavicular

(B) Posterior base

(C) Inferior vena cava

(D) Right mid-axillaries

58. Which of the following foods are highly suspect in anaphylaxis?

(A) Nuts

(B) Seafood

(C) Eggs

(D) Any food product may be involved in anaphylaxis

59. Which of the following is NOT a symptom of a heart attack?

(A) Chest pain

(B) Dyspnea

(C) Denial

(D) Headache

60. The beginning of obstetrical labor is the

(A) Discharge of the placenta.

(B) Fertilization of the ovum.

(C) Discharge of the cervical mucus plug.

(D) Rupture of the amniotic sack.

61. Which of the following drugs is useful in absorbing toxins in the stomach?

(A) Activated charcoal

(B) Ipecac

(C) Oxygen

(D) Aspirin

62. Labor concludes with

(A) The delivery of the baby.

(B) The delivery of the placenta.

(C) The delivery of the umbilical cord.

(D) The delivery of the amniotic fluid.

63. You are dispatched to a call for chest pains. You respond priority, the scene is safe and you are wearing protective equipment. Your patient is a female in her sixties, seated at the kitchen table. She is guarding her chest with one hand and tells you she has crushing chest pain of sudden onset. She has a history of cardiac problems and is currently on nitroglycerine paste and Cardizem™. Her pulse is weak and thready. Which of the following drugs should you not administer?

(A) Aspirin

(B) NTG

(C) Epinephrine

(D) Oxygen

KAPLAN

64. The preferred method of ventilating a patient in respiratory arrest in the prehospital setting is a

(A) Manual ventilator.
(B) Face mask.
(C) Bag valve mask.
(D) Bag valve mask with oxygen reservoir.

65. You are dispatched to a local restaurant for a man down. You arrive on scene and observe a male in full cardiac and respiratory arrest. You and your partner perform CPR for one minute and then convert his heart rhythm with the AED; he then has a pulse of 65 and a blood pressure of 90/60. After two minutes he begins to have spontaneous respirations and his gag reflex returns, so you remove the oropharyngeal airway. You finish your assessment and begin transport to the nearest emergency room 15 minutes away. At ten minutes from the hospital, he suddenly lapses into unconsciousness and again has no pulse or spontaneous respirations. Your next procedure should be

(A) Begin rescue breathing.
(B) Begin chest compressions.
(C) Analyze with the AED.
(D) Request an ALS intercept.

66. You are dispatched to a residence for an unconscious male. You respond priority with suitable precautions and the scene is safe. You find a male subject lying on the kitchen floor with spontaneous respirations, carotid and radial pulses. He is concious and responsive to verbal stimuli with a patent airway and no difficulty in swallowing. You take his blood sugar with a glucometer and he has a blood sugar of 30. He is probably suffering from

(A) Postictal seizure.
(B) Hypoglycemia.
(C) Hyperglycemia.
(D) Hypovolemia.

67. The patient in question 66 should be given

(A) Oxygen.
(B) Epinephrine.
(C) Glucose.
(D) Activase.

68. Presentation of the cord from the vagina before delivery of the baby is called

(A) Presenting cord.
(B) Prolapsed cord.
(C) Breech cord.
(D) Premature cord.

69. You are dispatched to a local clinic for a child convulsing. You respond priority wearing suitable precautions and arrive on scene. The nurse on scene advises that the mother brought her two-year-old male child in for not feeling well and as she began to examine him he began to seize. His vital signs are BP 100/60, pulse rate of 80, respirations of 18 prior to the seizure, and a rectal temperature of 105 degrees Fahrenheit. You suspect the patient is having a _____ seizure.

(A) Tonic/clonic
(B) Postictal
(C) Febrile
(D) Anaphylactic

70. Which of the following symptoms is NOT a symptom of a diabetic emergency?

(A) Impaired consciousness
(B) Fruity breath odor
(C) Mood changes
(D) Hypertension

71. Another term for heart attack is

(A) Myocardial infarction.
(B) Congestive Heart Failure.
(C) Mitral valve defect.
(D) Left bundle branch block.

72. You are dispatched to a call for a possible allergic reaction. You respond priority and arrive on scene, the scene is safe, and you are wearing suitable protective equipment. You are directed to a restaurant table where a male in his twenties is clutching his throat in severe respiratory distress. His partner tells you that he is allergic to nuts and nut products, but he has not had anything other than grilled steak with sautéed vegetables. Which drug do you want to administer following your initial assessment?

    (A) Ephedrine 5 mg tablet

    (B) Epinephrine 1:1000 .3mg intramuscular

    (C) Ephedrine spray sublingual

    (D) Oxygen 10-15 lpm via non-rebreather

73. Which of the following is NOT considered a toxin?

    (A) Poison ivy

    (B) Vodka

    (C) DDT

    (D) Hydrochlorothiazide

74. A motor vehicle accident in which one vehicle strikes another broadside is also referred to as a _____ crash.

    (A) Serious

    (B) Fatal

    (C) T-Bone

    (D) Bumper tapper

75. You are dispatched to a local residence for a female acting strangely. You respond priority wearing suitable precautions and arrive on scene simultaneously with the police. The house is extremely cold inside and the patient is a female in her sixties wearing heavy clothing. She responds to your questions in a faint intelligible voice and as you feel her neck for a carotid pulse she is cold to the touch. Your treatment of this patient should include all of the following except

    (A) Placing patient in a warm environment

    (B) Applying heat packs to the groin, axillary, and cervical regions

    (C) Advising the patient to drink rum

    (D) Removing wet clothing

76. The blood component that carries the antibodies the body uses to fight infection is (are) the

    (A) Hemoglobin.

    (B) Leukocytes.

    (C) Plasma.

    (D) Platelets.

77. You are dispatched to a residence for a patient unconscious. You respond priority and arrive on scene, the scene is safe, and you are wearing universal precautions. The firefighter on the scene advises that they have removed the victim from his garage where his car was running. The patient has labored breathing and his face is cyanotic, but his lips and tongue are bright red. Which poison should you suspect?

    (A) Carbon dioxide

    (B) Carbon monoxide

    (C) Gasoline

    (D) Narcotic overdose

78. Which of the following treatment facilities would you transport the patient in question 77 to?

    (A) Nearest Level One trauma center
    (B) Nearest emergency room
    (C) Nearest Level Three trauma center
    (D) Nearest facility with a hyperbaric chamber

79. On a very warm summer day you are dispatched to a road race site for a runner down. You respond priority and arrive on scene to find a 25 year old male lying unconscious on his back in his running clothes. He skin is red and dry and he is very hot to the touch. His pulse is 120, his respirations are 20, and his blood pressure is 100/60. Which condition should you suspect?

    (A) Heat cramps
    (B) Heat exhaustion
    (C) Heatstroke
    (D) Heat overdose

80. Which should you immediately do for the patient in question 79?

    (A) Transport priority
    (B) Request an ALS intercept
    (C) Administer oxygen 6 lpm via nasal cannula
    (D) Transfer the patient to a cooler location and apply wet cloths to his head

81. A phobia is

    (A) A feeling of sadness or worthlessness.
    (B) An alternate feeling of euphoria and depression.
    (C) An irrational fear.
    (D) A mistrust of everyone and everything.

82. Tuberculosis is an example of a(n) _____ pathogen.

    (A) Airborne
    (B) Bloodborne
    (C) Fluidborne
    (D) Still born

83. Which of the following poisons should not be vomited?

    (A) Bleach
    (B) Alcohol
    (C) Kerosene
    (D) Sodium hypochlorite

84. You are dispatched to a person in the water at a local reservoir. You respond priority and arrive on scene before the police and fire units and observe a male yelling for help 100 yards from shore. You should immediately

    (A) Jump into the water and swim to the victim.
    (B) Throw a life preserver to the victim.
    (C) Check and see if there is a boat nearby that you can use to row to the victim.
    (D) Advise dispatch that you will need a rescue boat.

85. The EMT should ask the patient to do which of the following prior to administration of a bronchodilator?

    (A) Hold their breath for five seconds
    (B) Exhale deeply
    (C) Inhale rapidly three times
    (D) Pant

86. Which of the following is NOT a poisonous sting or bite?

    (A) Bee sting
    (B) Black widow spider bite
    (C) Water moccasin snake bite
    (D) Dog bite

87. Which of the following behaviors constitutes a behavioral emergency?

    (A) Singing an inappropriate song on a city bus
    (B) Standing naked at a political fundraiser
    (C) Yelling obscenities at the scene of a motor vehicle accident
    (D) Threatening to commit suicide

88. Which of the following is not normally the cause for a behavioral emergency?

    (A) Head trauma

    (B) Hypoxia

    (C) Hypoglycemia

    (D) Hemoglobin

89. At which stage of hypothermia does loss of consciousness normally occur?

    (A) First stage

    (B) Second stage

    (C) Third stage

    (D) Fourth stage

90. Most behavioral emergency calls are

    (A) Violent

    (B) Nonviolent

    (C) Exaggerated

    (D) Wrongly dispatched

91. Which of the following is NOT considered a breech delivery?

    (A) Presentation of an arm or leg from the vagina

    (B) Presentation of the buttocks from the vagina

    (C) Presentation of the feet from the vagina

    (D) Presentation of the top of the head from the vagina

92. APGAR scores are taken at one minute and _____ _____ minutes post partum.

    (A) Two

    (B) Five

    (C) Ten

    (D) Twenty

93. The normal respiratory rate for an adult is

    (A) 6 to 12 times per minute

    (B) 12 to 20 times per minute

    (C) 15 to 25 times per minute

    (D) 20 to 40 times per minute

94. The heart contains _____ chambers.

    (A) One

    (B) Two

    (C) Three

    (D) Four

95. You are dispatched to a manufacturing plant for a worker complaining of difficulty breathing. You respond priority and arrive on scene wearing suitable precautions. The scene is safe. Your patient is a female in her fifties with a history of COPD. She is conscious, alert, and oriented times three complaining of dyspnea. Her vital signs are BP 180/100, pulse rate 92, respiratory rate 22, and pulse oximetry of 88 percent. Which of the following is a medication that may NOT be administered to this patient?

    (A) Oxygen

    (B) Albuterol

    (C) Epinephrine

    (D) Oral glucose

96. What is the minimum number of people required to safely restrain a violent patient in four point soft restraints.

    (A) Two

    (B) Three

    (C) Four

    (D) Five

97. In which of the following situations should a police escort be used?

    (A) Transport of a critical patient

    (B) Transport of a mother and child post partum

    (C) Unfamiliarity with the location of the hospital

    (D) Transport of a police officer injured in the line of duty

98. The normal gestation period for a human fetus is

    (A) 12 weeks
    (B) 24 weeks
    (C) 36 weeks
    (D) 52 weeks

99. The liquid component of the blood is called

    (A) Hemoglobin
    (B) Leukocytes
    (C) Plasma
    (D) Platelets

100. Obstetrical crowning is when

    (A) The mother's brow begins to perspire.
    (B) The baby's head becomes visible in the birth canal.
    (C) Labor pains are less than five minutes apart and last longer than one minute.
    (D) The baby cries for the first time.

101. Which of the following road conditions will most affect the stopping distance of an ambulance?

    (A) Wet roads
    (B) Roads under construction
    (C) Icy roads
    (D) Dry roads

102. A patient who exhibits multiple personalities during the assessment may be assumed to have

    (A) Bipolar disorder
    (B) Dissociative identity disorder
    (C) Manic-depressive syndrome
    (D) Panic disorder

103. You are dispatched to a call for a "possible heart attack" to a residence along with an ALS rescue that is ten minutes out. You respond priority and arrive on scene four minutes after being dispatched. The scene is safe and you are wearing appropriate universal precautions. You observe a male in his seventies lying supine on the living room floor, cyanotic, with his eyes open. You open his airway and note that he is not breathing. You administer two breaths, which inflate his lungs. You check for a carotid pulse and there is none. You advised your partner to begin chest compressions. What is your next step?

    (A) Continue rescue breathing and compressions pending arrival of ALS
    (B) Administer epinephrine 1:1000 1mg bolus
    (C) Apply the AED and follow the directions
    (D) After one minute of CPR, place the patient on a backboard and transport priority

104. Which of the following vehicles have the right of way over an ambulance?

    (A) Police cars with flashing lights operating
    (B) Fire trucks with flashing lights operating
    (C) School buses with flashing lights operating
    (D) Utility trucks with flashing yellow lights operating

105. The ulna is located in the

    (A) Lower arm.
    (B) Lower leg.
    (C) Chest.
    (D) Face.

106. You are dispatched to a woman in labor. You arrive on scene, the scene is safe, and you are wearing suitable precautions. You observe a woman in her twenties lying in bed with her knees drawn up and her upper body supported by pillows in a semi-Fowler position. She advises you that this is her third pregnancy, that her water has broken, and that the pains are less than a minute apart. You examine her vaginal area and as she experiences another contraction you see the top of the baby's head in the birth canal. You should next

(A) Prepare for immediate delivery.

(B) Place the mother on the stretcher left lateral recumbent and transport priority to the nearest obstetrical unit.

(C) Tie the mother's legs together to slow delivery while you do a full assessment.

(D) Boil water.

107. In the scenario in question 106, the next contraction delivers the baby's head. You notice the cord wrapped around the baby's neck. You should next

(A) Clamp the cord.

(B) Place two fingers between the cord and the baby's neck.

(C) Cut the cord.

(D) Request an ALS intercept.

108. In the scenario in question 106, after the baby is delivered you notice that she is not breathing. You should next

(A) Begin CPR.

(B) Suction with a bulb syringe.

(C) Suction with the portable suction unit.

(D) Slap the baby's bottom.

109. If a mistake is made in writing a PCR narrative, which of the following is correct?

(A) Disregard the error

(B) Destroy the document

(C) Cross out the error, write a correction, date and sign the correction

(D) Write a new narrative and staple it to the old narrative

110. Why are the bottom two ribs called floating ribs?

(A) They are not connected to the sternum

(B) They are not connected to any other bony structure

(C) They are suspended in fluid

(D) They are not really ribs

111. All calls for behavioral emergencies should also have a(n)

(A) ALS Intercept.

(B) Police response.

(C) Second rescue.

(D) Fire department response.

112. What is the maximum APGAR score?

(A) Five

(B) Eight

(C) Ten

(D) Twelve

113. The normal range for blood sugar levels is

(A) 30-60 mg/dl.

(B) 60-90 mg/dl.

(C) 80-120 mg/dl.

(D) 120-160 mg/dl.

114. Victims of sexual assault should be initially assessed and treated by

(A) EMTs of the same gender if possible.
(B) Police officers trained in sexual assault.
(C) Registered nurses.
(D) Rape crisis counselors.

115. Which of the following drugs will cause a patient to vomit violently?

(A) Oxygen
(B) Morphine
(C) Ipecac
(D) Activated charcoal

116. Which of the following incidents are the most common EMS trauma call?

(A) Falls
(B) Shootings
(C) Stabbings
(D) Motor vehicle accidents

117. In treatment of severe trauma, what is the recognized time standard from injury to the operating room?

(A) 30 minutes
(B) 60 minutes
(C) 180 minutes
(D) 240 minutes

118. The average human has how many quarts of blood in his or her circulatory system?

(A) Three
(B) Four
(C) Five
(D) Six

119. The most common cause of seizures in the infant population is

(A) Epilepsy.
(B) High fever.
(C) Poisoning.
(D) Mother's use of illegal drugs while pregnant.

120. You are dispatched to a residence for a man with a lacerated arm. You respond priority and arrive on scene wearing suitable precautions; police are on scene. Your patient is lying on the ground behind the house with a series of lacerations around his lower arm and is bleeding profusely. He is intoxicated and belligerent. You attempt to control the bleeding with pressure bandages but he continues to hemorrhage. Which procedure should be used next?

(A) Digital pressure
(B) Tourniquet
(C) MAST
(D) IV with Lactated Ringers

121. The most common cause of dyspnea in the infant is

(A) Foreign bodies.
(B) Mucus.
(C) Congenital birth defects.
(D) SIDS.

122. The difference between a dressing and a bandage is

(A) Size
(B) Shape
(C) Sterility
(D) Occlusiveness

123. Which of the following is not true as it pertains to refusal to treat or transport on the PCR?

    (A) The treatment and transport options must be explained.

    (B) The consequences of refusal must be explained.

    (C) The patient may not change their mind once they sign a refusal.

    (D) The signature of the patient must be witnessed by a disinterested third party.

124. You are dispatched to a motor vehicle accident on the highway. You respond priority and arrive on scene wearing suitable BSI gear. The police and fire department are on scene. Your patient is a male lying next to his wrecked car. He has been collared and spineboarded by the fire department. He is responsive to painful stimuli with vital signs of BP 100/60, pulse of 120, respirations of 18. He is pale and clammy. Your treatment of this patient should include all of the following except

    (A) Trendelenburg position.

    (B) Prevention of heat loss.

    (C) High flow oxygen.

    (D) Fowler position.

125. Which of the following is not a type of open wound?

    (A) Abrasion

    (B) Incision

    (C) Bruising

    (D) Laceration

126. One of the side effects of nitroglycerin tablets is

    (A) Hypotension

    (B) Hypertension

    (C) Headache

    (D) Cerebral hemorrhage

127. Wounds to which of the following anatomical areas should be treated with occlusive dressings?

    (A) Head

    (B) Neck

    (C) Abdomen

    (D) Genitals

128. You are dispatched along with the fire department to a report of a person on fire behind a residence. You respond priority and arrive simultaneously with the fire department. A woman tells you her husband was lighting his charcoal grill with gasoline and there was an explosion. The patient is a male subject who is conscious, alert, and oriented times three. He states he was trying to light the grill when the gasoline exploded. He denies any dyspnea. The physical exam reveals second degree burns to both arms and there is no other part of the body burnt. What percentage of the patient's body is burnt?

    (A) Nine percent

    (B) Eighteen percent

    (C) Twenty seven percent

    (D) Twenty percent

129. In the scenario in question 128 what priority is this patient?

    (A) Nonpriority

    (B) Moderate

    (C) Critical

    (D) Fatal

130. Electrical burns may be complicated by

    (A) Scene safety concerns

    (B) Respiratory distress

    (C) Cardiac dysrhythmias

    (D) Increased risk of infection

131. You are dispatched to the high school football field for a player injured. You respond priority and arrive on scene wearing suitable precautions. The trainer advises you he suspects the player has a fractured fibula. The patient is conscious, alert, and oriented times three and his only complaint is severe pain in his lower leg. When considering what type of splint you are going to apply you must always splint the suspected fracture site and

(A) The inferior joint.
(B) The adjacent joints.
(C) The adjacent bone.
(D) The superior joint.

132. In the scenario in question 131, which situation would lead you to attempt to reduce the broken bone?

(A) Lower leg fracture
(B) Absence of distal pulse
(C) Hypovolemic shock
(D) Femur fracture

133. The letter "M" in the acronym SAMPLE stands for

(A) Menstrual period.
(B) Medications.
(C) Most active symptom.
(D) Morning routine.

134. The epiglottis in a pediatric patient is _____ in the airway than in an adult patient.

(A) More sensitive
(B) Higher
(C) Lower
(D) More anterior

135. In which of the following injury situations should you apply a cervical collar?

(A) Head trauma secondary to a rear end motor vehicle collision
(B) Fall from a garage roof
(C) Neck pain as a result of sleeping in a wrong position
(D) All of the above

136. The narrative section of the prehospital care report should include all of the following except

(A) What the patient looked like on EMS arrival.
(B) What medications the patient is currently taking.
(C) The vital signs of the patient.
(D) The patient's next of kin

137. You are dispatched to a two-car motor vehicle accident and respond priority. You arrive on scene, the scene is safe, and you are wearing appropriate precautions. Your patient is in a vehicle that was struck broadside by another vehicle traveling at a high rate of speed. He was not restrained and is complaining of dyspnea. His shirt is ripped and bloody and you notice that he has an open wound that is gurgling and foaming. This patient is most at risk for

(A) Hypovolemic shock.
(B) Pneumothorax.
(C) Subdural hematoma.
(D) Congestive heart failure.

138. Patients with open abdominal injuries are at a greater risk for

(A) Hypotension.
(B) Infection.
(C) Sudden cardiac death.
(D) Lawsuits.

139. A patient aged eight months is defined as a

   (A) Neonate.

   (B) Toddler.

   (C) Infant.

   (D) Preschooler.

140. If a tourniquet is applied to control bleeding, at what point should it be loosened?

   (A) Every five minutes

   (B) Every ten minutes

   (C) Every fifteen minutes

   (D) At the hospital

141. You respond along with police to a local residence for a psychological evaluation. You respond priority with suitable precautions and when you arrive the police have secured the scene. Your patient is a male in his thirties pacing around the room anxiously. He is not cooperative or responsive to your questions and the police advise that his psychiatrist is requesting that he be transported to the nearest emergency room for medical evaluation prior to admittance to the psychiatric facility. As the patient hears this he attacks the police officer, but is quickly subdued. The police officer advises you that his psychiatrist has approved the use of restraints. What is the most proper way to restrain this patient?

   (A) Prone with hands behind the back and ankles drawn up to the wrists

   (B) Supine with hands behind the back and ankles secured to the stretcher

   (C) Supine with hands in front and secured to the abdomen and ankles secured to the stretcher

   (D) Prone between two backboards locked together with handcuffs

142. You are dispatched to a local nursing home for a patient who has fallen. You respond priority with suitable precautions and the scene is safe. You find an 82-year-old female lying supine on the floor, conscious and alert, complaining of pain to her hip. You note that her right leg is rotated outward. What splinting device should you use?

   (A) Traction splint

   (B) Air splint

   (C) Velcro splint

   (D) Backboard

143. Which of the following types of bleeding is the most severe?

   (A) Capillary

   (B) Venous

   (C) Arteriole

   (D) Arterial

144. Aspirin is indicated for which of the following conditions in EMS protocols?

   (A) Headache

   (B) Chest pain

   (C) Abdominal pain

   (D) Leg and arm pain

145. Which of the following persons are not allowed to routinely access a prehospital care report?

   (A) The patient

   (B) The receiving physician

   (C) The police

   (D) The EMT who wrote the report

146. Improper use of restraints can lead to all of the following except

   (A) Death of a patient.

   (B) Arrest of an EMT.

   (C) Injury to the patient.

   (D) Scene safety.

147. Which of the following pregnancies will normally have a longer labor period?

    (A) First
    (B) Second
    (C) Third
    (D) Fourth

148. At the scene of a motor vehicle accident, the ambulance should be parked so as to

    (A) Be readily accessible.
    (B) Protect the scene.
    (C) Be able to load the patient into the back doors.
    (D) Not obstruct the police investigation.

149. Once the cervix is fully dilated and the baby "drops" into the birth canal, this is referred to as

    (A) First stage labor.
    (B) Second stage labor.
    (C) Third stage labor.
    (D) Fourth stage labor.

150. Which of the following is an example of implied consent?

    (A) Patient who agrees to be transported to the emergency room
    (B) Pediatric patient whose parent allows him to be treated and transported
    (C) Unconscious patient
    (D) Patient who is diagnosed with schizophrenia and refuses transport

ANSWER KEY ON FOLLOWING PAGE

Practice Test: **Answer Key**

1. C	31. A	61. A	91. D	121. B
2. C	32. B	62. B	92. B	122. C
3. D	33. B	63. C	93. B	123. D
4. C	34. A	64. D	94. D	124. D
5. D	35. C	65. A	95. D	125. C
6. D	36. A	66. B	96. D	126. A
7. C	37. D	67. C	97. C	127. B
8. D	38. B	68. B	98. C	128. B
9. D	39. C	69. C	99. C	129. C
10. D	40. D	70. D	100. B	130. C
11. C	41. C	71. A	101. C	131. B
12. D	42. D	72. B	102. B	132. B
13. A	43. B	73. D	103. C	133. B
14. D	44. A	74. C	104. C	134. B
15. B	45. B	75. C	105. A	135. D
16. C	46. D	76. B	106. A	136. D
17. D	47. D	77. B	107. B	137. B
18. C	48. B	78. D	108. B	138. B
19. A	49. A	79. C	109. C	139. C
20. B	50. C	80. D	110. A	140. D
21. C	51. D	81. C	111. B	141. C
22. D	52. C	82. A	112. C	142. D
23. D	53. A	83. C	113. C	143. D
24. D	54. B	84. C	114. A	144. B
25. A	55. D	85. B	115. C	145. C
26. D	56. C	86. D	116. D	146. D
27. A	57. C	87. D	117. B	147. A
28. C	58. D	88. D	118. B	148. B
29. B	59. D	89. C	119. B	149. B
30. B	60. C	90. B	120. A	150. C

Practice Test Answers and Explanations

1. C

Any dispatch to a call with violence involved, such as a gunshot wound, must be secured by police prior to EMS involvement. The other calls do not give any indication of being unsafe.

2. C

The path of blood flow goes from the heart to the aorta to the arteries to the arterioles to the capillaries to the venules to the veins to the vena cavae to the heart.

3. D

The very young and very old are at greater risk for hypothermia.

4. C

Crying may be a response to the depressive stage of grief, but is not itself a stage of grief. The other answers are all among the five stages. The other two are depression and bargaining.

5. D

The zygomatic bones are the cheekbones.

6. D

A minor is legally unable to give consent. A person who is unconscious likewise cannot give expressed consent but may be treated under the doctrine of implied consent. A mentally challenged person cannot give legal consent either. Answer (D) is correct because the patient is of the legal age of majority and has no indications that she is incompetent to give or refuse consent.

7. C

Helicopters are dangerous vehicles, and safety rules include never approaching from the uphill side because of the danger of the rotors, or from the rear because of the tail rotor. In addition, EMTs should never approach until instructed by a helicopter crew member so that the patient loading can be coordinated safely. Not approaching the helicopter at all may be impractical due to patient care concerns.

8. D

(A), (B), and (C) are all significant in conducting patient assessment. A patient's medical insurance is not a consideration in treating emergency patients.

9. D

(A), (B), and (C) are all components of the Glasgow Coma Scale.

10. D

An EMT-Basic must protect a patient's confidentiality; however, the legal statutes do require that certain parties be notified of those conditions listed in (A), (B), and (C). There is no requirement, however, to notify the authorities of a patient's history of treatment for AIDS, and such disclosure may place the EMT at risk for legal actions.

11. C

Superior refers to an upper region, so the head is considered superior to the chest, while the chest would be considered inferior to the head. Anterior is the front, and posterior is the back.

12. D

The head, torso, and extremities are all checked in a head-to-toe trauma assessment. The genitals are checked visually for trauma, discharge, and priapism (erection) in the male.

13. A

The cervical section of the spine has 7, the thoracic 12, the lumbar 5, the sacral 5, and the coccyx 4.

14. D

Loss of spontaneity is not a characteristic symptom of post-traumatic stress disorder. The other answers are all symptoms of PTSD, and if they last longer then a few days, the EMT-Basic should be referred for professional help.

15. B

The baby's ability to make facial expressions is indicative of its ability to function in the outside world. Grating refers to rubbing of two organs together, guarding is when one protects a portion of the body with one's hands, and gurgling is the sound one makes when there is fluid in the oropharynx. None of these are indicators in the APGAR score.

16. C

Unless contraindicated by some other condition, women in their third trimester of pregnancy should be transported on their left side to prevent the weight of the child from compressing their vena cavae and causing circulatory problems, which could lead to impairment of consciousness and other complications. Trendelenburg is when the legs are elevated to help combat hypotension, and Fowler position is seated upright.

17. D

Those most at risk for suicide are males over the age of 40 who are single, widowed, or divorced with a history of alcohol or drug abuse and depression; those with a defined lethal plan that they will verbalize; those who have an unusual gathering of objects that can cause death; those with a previous history of suicidal behavior; people with a recent diagnosis of serious illness, recent loss of a significant loved one, or recent loss of a job; and people who have been arrested or sentenced to imprisonment. Bankruptcy has not been identified as a condition that places people at greater risk for suicide.

18. C

The patient is not exhibiting a behavior that requires you to respond with overly aggressive technique, such as tackling her or wrestling her to the stretcher. She is having delusions, and it is not wise to give these delusions credence by acknowledging them, such as by shaking Mr. Nureyev's hand. She might protest when you tell her that Mr. Nureyev is not right there dancing with her, but your confidence and gentle demeanor will more often than not win her over to doing what you would like her to do.

19. A

Neonates have higher pulse rates and respiratory rates than infants. There is no change in regularity between neonates and infants.

20. B

Most EMTs are injured while treating injured patients at motor vehicle accidents and thus should be more alert to the dangers posed by being on the streets and highways. The other situations also present dangers of which the EMT must be aware, but the MVA is the leading cause of injury.

21. C

Veins carry blood toward the heart. The vessels that carry blood away from the heart are the arteries.

22. D

The three types of muscles are voluntary, involuntary, and cardiac. There is no such thing as a regulatory muscle.

23. D

SAMPLE stands for Signs and symptoms, Allergies, Medications, Pertinent past history, Last oral intake, and Events leading up to this situation. Pulse rate is a vital sign.

24. D

Communications equipment should be checked at the start of each shift. No self-respecting EMT-Basic would like to find out two hours into the shift that his radio was not working and that calls were missed.

25. A

Before anything else is done, the EMT-Basic must be certain that the scene is safe to operate in. Universal precautions should already be in place prior to arrival on scene, and only then should patient assessment begin with checking the airway.

26. D

There is no legal limit for declaring that a person is so impaired as to be judged incompetent. It is a judgment call on the part of the EMT-Basic.

27. A

Once the scene is determined to be safe and the EMT is wearing proper precautions, she must assure that the patient has a patent airway.

28. C

Answers (A), (B), and (D) are all descriptions of levels of consciousness.

29. B

Perfusion refers to the percentage of oxygen that a red blood cell can carry to the cells and is measured by the use of the pulse oximeter. This is a vital sign for determining how efficiently the lungs are transferring oxygen to the red blood cells and how well the heart is pumping those cells throughout the body. Basic EMS does not have the diagnostic capabilities to determine the other answers.

30. B

Hypothermic means low temperature. The prefix *hypo-* means "below," and the root *thermia* refers to temperature; clinically, hypothermia means "below normal temperature." Too hot would be "hyperthermia," too sweaty would be "diaphoretic," and too dry would be "arid."

31. A

This patient may benefit from an ALS intervention depending on his underlying medical problem. Since ALS is within half the time that it would take to get him to an emergency room, this would be the most correct solution. The administration of epinephrine would be used only if the assessment gave some indication that his level of consciousness was due to an allergic reaction. The helicopter is not really appropriate in this situation since the amount of time spent taking off and landing would delay arrival of the patient at the emergency room.

32. B

OPQRST stands for **O**nset, **P**rovocation, **Q**uality, **R**adiation, **S**everity, and **T**ime. This question also reinforces the need to read the question carefully, since the words "quality" and "quantity" are very close.

33. B

Good patient assessment requires that vital signs and assessment observations be checked and trended every five minutes.

34. A

While the other answers all are potentially serious, a fall from more than 20 feet definitely requires an immediate transport. A bicycle accident would be considered "load and go" if the victim were under the age of 12.

35. C

The mnemonic DCAP-BTLS is used in the focused assessment of a trauma patient and stands for **D**eformity, **C**ontusions, **A**brasions, **P**unctures, **B**urns, **T**enderness, **L**acerations, and **S**welling.

36. A

The midaxillary line runs through the underarm of the patient, dividing the anterior plane from the posterior plane.

37. D

This is the type of question that challenges your knowledge. The tendency is to choose one of the "H" answers since the correct answer seems out of place, and there is such a thing as the Hare Traction Splint.

38. B

The Good Samaritan Act was passed to encourage people to render aid by minimizing the liability for such acts.

39. C

While five minutes is the standard, vital signs should be retaken anytime there is any change in the patient's condition. Changes in the patient's condition will only be noted if the patient's ongoing assessment is constant and not just at a predetermined interval.

40. D

AVPU stands for **A**lert, **V**erbal, **P**ain, **U**nresponsive, and is used to assign a level of consciousness to a patient. A patient who does not awaken when yelled at, and doesn't respond to a vigorous rubbing of his sternum is considered **U**nresponsive to pain.

41. C

Patient confidentiality laws mandate that the patient's name and specific medical information be kept confidential. Broadcasting a patient's name over the radio, which is monitored, would be a violation of this confidentiality. (A) and (B) would be important information in responding to a call.

42. D

While some reports do have spaces for medical insurance information for use by billing services, this information is not required for the patient care report.

43. B

When bandaging an eye injury, you must cover both eyes to prevent the sympathetic movement of the uninjured eye from causing further injury to the injured eye. Without any other injuries, there is no need to bandage the entire upper head.

44. A

All states mandate reporting by medical providers to the appropriate state agency if they become aware of child abuse. Some states also require reporting of sexual abuse, elder abuse, and spousal abuse, but this not yet universal.

45. B

Once the cord ceases pulsing and the baby is breathing on his or her own, it is safe to cut the cord. If the cord is cut before the pulsing has ceased, there is a danger of the mother exsanguinating (bleeding). In waiting until the placenta is delivered, there is no increased danger to the mother or neonate, nor would waiting to arrive at the hospital be a problem, however, in order to properly treat the neonate, it would be easier to have him or her separated from the placenta.

46. D

Dropping blood pressure, excessive thirst, and tachypnea are all symptoms of hypovolemic shock, along with tachycardia, or fast heart rate. Bradycardia is a slow heart rate.

47. D

A competent and conscious patient may refuse any medical procedure or transport.

48. B

Oxygen is normally inhaled into the lungs by the breathing action of the patient. Liquid substances may be taken orally or injected, and certain medications are most effective when placed under the tongue, or sublingually.

49. A

SIDS normally occurs in the neonate and infant populations, although toddlers are also occasionally at risk.

50. C

An impaled object should never be removed to keep bleeding under control, unless it interferes with managing the airway or performing chest compressions.

51. D

The expiration date must always be checked. The other answers should also be checked, but answer (D), right date, is one of the "Five Rights" to be checked in drug administration.

52. C

Tripod position is when a patient is seated leaning forward, with his or her shoulders rotated outward to allow for less effort on inspiration. Semi-Fowler is a supine position at a 45-degree angle, and supine is merely lying flat on one's back.

53. A

The systolic pressure in the arteries occurs when the ventricles contract and force the blood through the circulatory system. Diastolic pressure occurs when the heart is relaxing between contractions. Arterial pressure is the general pressure in the arteries.

54. B

The patient may still be resuscitated, since his vital signs may have been suppressed by sudden immersion in cold water, a condition referred to as the mammalian diving reflex. EMS personnel cannot normally pronounce people dead, although state protocols do usually allow EMTs to assume death has occurred if certain signs and symptoms, such as rigor mortis and postmortem lividity, are present. You will want to warm the patient by cutting away his clothing and placing him in a warm truck, but your priority should be beginning CPR. You may request an ALS intercept, but it is imperative that Basic Life Support begin immediately.

55. D

The patient is hypoxic and needs high-flow oxygen, and the device that will provide the most flow is the full non-rebreather, which delivers between 80 and 100 percent oxygen to the patient. The other devices deliver less: the nasal cannula delivers 20 to 40 percent, the simple face mask 40 to 60 percent, and the partial nonrebreather 60 to 80 percent.

56. C

The maximum liter flow for the full nonrebreather is 15 liters per minute.

57. C

The inferior vena cava is a blood vessel that returns deoxygenated blood to the heart and has little to do with auscultation of breath sounds.

58. D

Any food product may be implicated in anaphylaxis, or allergic reaction.

59. D

All of the other answers, including denial, are symptoms of a myocardial infarction.

60. C

The first stage of labor begins when the mucus plug is discharged from the cervix. Labor ends following the delivery of the placenta, or afterbirth. Fertilization of the ovum is the beginning of gestation or pregnancy. The amniotic sac usually, but not always, ruptures during the first stage of labor after the mucus plug is discharged.

61. A

Activated charcoal is very effective at absorbing toxins in the stomach before they can be absorbed into the bloodstream. Ipecac causes vomiting, oxygen is used for respiratory problems, and aspirin is an analgesic and in EMS is used only in the chest pain protocols.

62. B

Labor concludes with the delivery of the placenta.

63. C

Epinephrine is indicated in cardiac arrest, but not in the treatment of chest pain, nor is it in most BLS protocols. Oxygen and aspirin are always indicated in the treatment of sudden chest pain. Medical control may order nitroglycerin if state protocols allow.

64. D

A BVM with an oxygen reservoir is the most effective method of ventilating a patient in the prehospital setting. A manual ventilator is unwieldy in the prehospital, setting and a face mask is not as effective in ventilating as a bag-valve mask. The oxygen reservoir also makes the delivery of oxygen much higher than the other prehospital devices do.

65. A

The sequence for a second resuscitation following an arrest is identical: ABC (airway, breathing, and circulation), then AED. ALS intercept is also a possibility, but the best answer is airway.

66. B

This patient is having a diabetic emergency caused by low blood sugar, or hypoglycemia. Normal blood sugar is 80 to 120. Postictal seizure meets the symptoms except for the low blood sugar; hyperglycemia is high blood sugar, which is definitely not the case here; and hypovolemia would be caused by loss of blood volume, of which there's no indication in the signs given in the question.

67. C

The patient's blood sugar must be elevated. This is done by administering sugar, or glucose. Oxygen would be indicated if oxygen perfusion were low, epinephrine for allergic reaction, and nitroglycerin for chest pain.

68. B

When the cord presents first, there is great danger that the cord will be compressed between the vaginal walls and the baby's head, cutting off circulation and oxygen to the baby. This is also technically a breech delivery, but "prolapsed cord" is the more correct terminology.

69. C

Most infant seizures are caused by a high temperature, or fever. Tonic/clonic refers to the extremely jerky movements of a full-blown seizure, postictal is the state of unconsciousness that follows the tonic/clonic portion of the seizure, and anaphylactic refers to allergic reaction.

70. D

High blood pressure is not a symptom of a diabetic emergency; however, impaired consciousness, fruity breath odors, and mood changes are all indicative of this condition.

71. A

A heart attack occurs when a coronary artery is blocked and in turn a portion of the heart muscle becomes ischemic from lack of oxygen, or infarcts. The other answers are all cardiac conditions, but not literally a heart attack.

72. B

This patient is exhibiting symptoms of an allergic reaction and needs the immediate intervention of epinephrine, an intervention allowed by many state protocols. Even if he has not knowingly ingested any known allergen, the food he has eaten may have been prepared with a nut product and this may be the cause. Ephredrine is an ingredient in cough syrup and is not used in EMS. NTG is for chest pain. Oxygen may be indicated, but epinephrine is the better answer.

73. D

Poison ivy, vodka, and DDT are toxins or poisons if contacted or consumed in unsafe quantities. HCTZ is a drug used in the treatment of hypertension.

74. C

A vehicle struck broadside is referred to as a T-bone crash. All these crashes may be serious or fatal, but the best answer is T-bone.

75. C

The giving of alcohol to a hypothermic patient is an old wives' tale and will actually decrease the body's ability to respond to the cold and cause a more rapid descent into the higher stages of hypothermia. The other answers are all appropriate treatments of hypothermia.

76. B

Leukocytes, or white blood cells, are the body's primary mechanism in combating infection and disease.

77. B

The telltale sign of carbon-monoxide poisoning is bright red lips and tongue. Carbon dioxide is not directly poisonous but can cause anoxia, since it displaces oxygen in the air; gasoline is a petroleum distillate; and a narcotic overdose will not cause red lips.

78. D

Carbon-monoxide poisoning is best treated by a hyperbaric chamber. Such a chamber forces oxygen into the hemoglobin under pressure and displaces the carbon monoxide. State protocols and medical control naturally dictate the proper course of action. A Level One trauma center has equipment and staff to deal with all cases of trauma, while a Level Three center has minimal equipment and staff and will often stabilize a patient in preparation for transfer to a Level One center.

79. C

The patient's condition indicates that his sweating mechanism has been compromised and his temperature is dangerously high. This condition is called heatstroke. Heat cramps are muscle aches caused by hyperthermia, and heat exhaustion is impaired consciousness brought on by hyperthermia, but without the disruption of the sweating mechanism.

80. D

This patient needs to be cooled immediately and then transported. Oxygen and an ALS intercept are also possibilities, but the priority has to be to get the patient cooled down to prevent seizures, possible brain insult, and death.

81. C

Phobias are irrational fears. A feeling of sadness or worthlessness is often the result of clinical depression, the alternating feelings of euphoria and depression are symptomatic of bipolar disorder, and a mistrust of everyone and everything is paranoia.

82. A

Tuberculosis is transmitted by an airborne bacteria.

83. C

Petroleum products, such as kerosene, should never be vomited back up, as there is the danger of aspiration of the petroleum into the lungs. Bleach and sodium hypochloride are the same thing and may be vomited.

84. C

The victim is too far to reach with a life preserver, and you should never attempt to swim to a victim unless you are confident in your own swimming ability and in your ability to actually rescue a drowning person. If there is no boat, then you will want to notify dispatch to send one.

85. B

Prior to the administration of a bronchodilator, the EMT-Basic asks the patient to exhale deeply to remove as much air from the lungs as possible, and then to inhale the vapor deeply into the lungs for maximum effect.

86. D

All of the bites and stings listed except for the dog bite could be toxic. Dog bites may present other problems, including rabies, but are not generally considered toxic

87. D

Threatening to kill oneself or someone else constitutes a behavior emergency and requires immediate intervention. Answer choices (A) and (B) may be disturbing or illegal, but by themselves do not constitute probable cause for EMS intervention. Yelling obscenities at a motor vehicle accident is not nice, but is a relatively normal response. Verbalizing suicide or homicide are words that permit public safety personnel to intervene.

88. D

Hemoglobin, or red blood cells, carries oxygen in the circulatory system. The other answers are all possible causes of improper behaviors that constitute a behavioral emergency.

89. C

Unconsciousness usually occurs in the third stage of hypothermia. First-stage hypothermia is marked by shivering as the body tries to raise its temperature. The second stage is when consciousness and judgment begin to become impaired and there is a loss of motor functions. In the third stage, unconsciousness sets in and the extremities begin to freeze. The fourth stage of hypothermia is marked by decreasing vital signs, and in the fifth stage, death occurs.

90. B

Most behavioral emergency calls are nonviolent, but the EMT must always be prepared to deal with violent patients.

91. D

A breech birth is defined as the first presentation of any part of the baby other than the head.

92. B

APGAR scores are taken at one and five minutes post partum.

93. B

Most texts give the normal adult respiratory rate as 12 to 20 times per minute. None of the other answers would be considered normal.

94. D

The four chambers are the left and right atria and the left and right ventricles.

95. D

The first three medications may be administered for dyspnea, although the use of albuterol and epinephrine are dependent on state protocols and medical control. Oral glucose is indicated for hypoglycemia or low blood sugar

96. D

Five people are needed: one person for each limb and one to apply the restraints.

97. C

The use of police escorts has been shown to be more dangerous than not having one. Therefore, the only time one should be used is when the ambulance crew is uncertain of the route to the hospital.

98. C

The normal gestation period is nine months from conception, or 36 weeks.

99. C

Plasma is the liquid part of the blood that carries the other components through the circulatory system. The other components are hemoglobin, or red blood cells; leukocytes or white blood cells; and platelets.

100. B

Crowning is when the baby's head becomes visible. The mother's perspiration and the baby's crying have nothing to do with this term. When pains are less than five minutes apart and last longer than one minute, this usually indicates that delivery is imminent.

101. C

Icy roads are the most slippery of the four.

102. B

Dissociative identity disorder can be seen when a patient presents with multiple personalities; such individuals may have been victims of severe abuse. Bipolar disorder is the same as manic-depressive syndrome; symptoms are feelings that change from extreme euphoria to extreme depression. Panic disorder is when the patient becomes overly anxious about a situation that does not warrant that sort of response.

103. C

Application of the AED may diagnose a dysrhythmia, which may then be treated by a countershock and restore a normal heartbeat, or it may advise to continue CPR. Administration of epinephrine in this instance is an ALS intervention and since ALS has already been dispatched, you should maintain your patient with CPR pending their arrival, but your first step is to apply the AED.

104. C

School buses with flashing lights have the right of way over all other vehicles, including ambulances. Police cars and fire trucks have the same rights of way as ambulances, but no additional privileges.

105. A

The ulna is one of the two bones in the lower arm.

106. A

Crowning is indicative of imminent delivery. Attempting to transport the mother at this point will result in delivery in the back of the ambulance. The legs should never be tied together, as this will cause damage to both the mother and the baby. Boiling water is what you send the new father to get to keep him out of the way.

107. B

If the baby presents with the cord wrapped around the neck, you must either unwrap the cord or open the baby's airway by relieving the pressure of the cord around the neck. Clamping or cutting the cord will impair the circulation of the baby and may cause the mother to bleed out.

108. B

Immediately after delivery, the baby's mouth and nose should be suctioned with a bulb syringe to facilitate the baby's own breathing. A portable suction unit provides too much suction and could damage the baby's lungs. Slapping the baby's bottom may help stimulate spontaneous respirations, but you still need to clear the airway first. If the baby does not start breathing spontaneously, then begin CPR.

109. C

A PCR is a legal document, and changes may only be made by the person writing the actual narrative. The changes must be noticeable and documented, and are best made by writing a single line through the error and by initialing and dating the change. Disregarding the error would compound the error by making it appear that it was the actual assessment noted or treatment given. Destroying the document would break the serial change of reports required for authenticity, and writing a new narrative and stapling it to the old would cause confusion as to which narrative was correct, especially if the forms became separated.

110. A

The bottom two ribs are not connected to the sternum and are called floating ribs. The other ribs are all connected to both the sternum and the vertebrae.

111. B

While most behavioral calls are nonviolent, the potential for violence exists and warrants police presence. ALS units may have the ability to administer sedatives to violent patients, and might be included, but police would still be necessary. A second rescue or the fire department would only be necessary if more manpower was necessary to restrain the patient, if indicated.

112. C

Either 1 or 2 points are given for each element of the APGAR score, for a maximum of 10.

113. C

Most texts give 80–120 mg/dl as normal. Answer choices (A) and (B) would be considered hypoglycemia, and answer choice (D) would be considered mild hyperglycemia.

114. A

Victims of a sexual assault may be suspicious of EMTs of the same gender as their attacker, and might prefer to share sensitive information with an EMT of their own gender. Police officers and rape crisis counselors are important in the follow-up treatment of these victims, as are registered nurses, but initial prehospital care should be done by an EMT, preferably one of the same gender.

115. C

Ipecac may be ordered by medical control to cause a patient to vomit his or her stomach contents if medical control feels that would be the best course of treatment in a poisoning or overdose situation. Morphine and activated charcoal may also cause vomiting as side effects, but the purpose of ipecac is precisely that of an emetic, making it the better answer.

116. D

The most common EMS trauma call is for motor vehicle accidents.

117. B

Numerous studies have shown that survivability increases dramatically if a patient with severe trauma can have surgical intervention within the Golden Hour, or 60 minutes.

118. B

The average adult human has four quarts of blood.

119. B

A high temperature is the most frequent cause of pediatric seizures, followed by epilepsy, poisoning, and drug exposure to the fetus while in the mother's uterus.

120. A

The correct sequence of attempting to control severe bleeding is direct pressure, digital pressure, and a tourniquet as a last resort. An IV with Lactated Ringers has nothing to do with controlling hemorrhage.

121. B

Since infants are nose-breathers, upper respiratory infections cause mucus buildup, which causes difficulty breathing in the neonate and infant population. Foreign bodies and birth defects can also cause dyspnea, but mucus is the most common cause. Sudden Infant Death Syndrome refers to a condition where a previously healthy infant is found dead with no explicable cause.

122. C

A dressing is always sterile and may be of any size or shape. A special type of dressing is called occlusive, which blocks air from entering the wound and is used for wounds near airways in the chest and neck.

123. C

A patient may always change his or her mind, even after signing a refusal. When a patient refuses treatment or transport, all options must be explained as well as the possible medical consequences. The signature of the patient on the refusal form should be witnessed by a disinterested third party to attest to the facts of the refusal.

KAPLAN

124. D

Trendelenburg position, the raising of the feet above the head, retaining body heat, and administration of oxygen are all treatments for shock. Fowler position is seated upright and is not indicated for treatment of hypovolemia.

125. C

Bruising is a type of closed wound; the skin is not open to the outside. Abrasions, incisions, and lacerations are all types of open wounds.

126. A

NTG (nitroglycerin) is a potent vasodilator, which accounts for its effectiveness in relieving chest pain caused by reduced blood flow in the carotid arteries. It consequently may lead to lowered blood pressure, or hypotension. It may also cause headache, but hypotension is the more common side effect and the better answer.

127. B

A wound in the neck that may leak air into the body should be dressed with an occlusive dressing to keep air from entering and contributing to a pneumothorax. Wounds to the genitals, head, and abdomen may be dressed with ordinary dressings.

128. B

By the rule of nines, each arm is 9 percent of body surface, so both arms would be a total of 18 percent.

129. C

Second-degree, or partial-thickness, burns are critical if they involve an entire body part. Normally a second-degree burn would be considered critical only if it involved more than 30 percent of body area.

130. C

Electrical injuries may interrupt the electrical activity of the heart and cause cardiac dysrhythmias. Scene safety, respiratory distress, and increased risk of infection are all concerns of burn injuries, but the best answer is the one that involves the heart.

131. B

A properly applied splint always secures the broken bone and both adjacent joints, not just one adjacent joint.

132. B

If a fracture occludes the artery feeding the distal portion of the extremity, then the cells will die and amputation becomes a real possibility. The goal in realigning the bone is to restore circulation to the extremity. The other fractures should be splinted as they are found.

133. B

SAMPLE stands for **S**igns and **s**ymptoms, **A**llergies, **M**edications, **P**ast history, **L**ast oral intake, and **E**vents leading up to the situation.

134. B

The epiglottis is higher in the airway of an infant, an important anatomical difference.

135. D

Cervical spine injury should be considered in all trauma situations unless you can definitely rule it out. Neck pain brought about by sleeping also calls for immobilization until damage to the spinal cord can be ruled out.

136. D

(A), (B), and (C) are all necessary to the narrative, both to document what the EMT-Basic assessed about the patient for legal purposes and to assist the receiving physician in making his or her diagnosis.

137. B

The foaming of a wound to the chest indicates that the pleural cavity has been compromised; as the air pressure builds in the pleural space, the lung will not be able to expand normally. This condition is referred to as a pneumothorax.

138. B

Abdominal wounds are at a high risk for infection if the contents of the gastrointestinal tract spill into the abdominal compartment. Hypotension and sudden cardiac death are always a possibility in serious injuries, as are lawsuits, but the best answer is infection.

139. C

Neonates are aged from birth to four weeks, infants from four weeks to one year, toddlers from one to three years, preschoolers from 3 to 6 years, school-age children from 6 to 12 years, and adolescents from 12 to 18 years of age.

140. D

A tourniquet once applied should never be released in the field since serious shock may develop; therefore, it should only be released once the patient is in the hospital and bleeding may be controlled surgically.

141. C

Four-point restraints require that each limb be restrained. The patient should always be supine so that you can intervene immediately if it becomes necessary to intervene for another medical condition, such as cardiac arrest. Patients should never be restrained facedown, as it causes pressure on the diaphragm that may lead to apnea and sudden death, which may not be apparent if the patient is facedown. Likewise, the patient should never be made to lie on his restrained limbs due to the risk of impaired circulation in the extremities.

142. D

In order to properly immobilize a fractured hip, the patient must be secured to a long spineboard. The other splints would not do this.

143. D

A lacerated artery will bleed more readily due to the higher pressure in the arteries, as well as due to the pulsing action that makes clotting more difficult. Arterioles are smaller arteries and will clot more readily than a larger vessel, and veins and capillaries flow at lower pressures that facilitate clotting.

144. B

Aspirin is given for chest pain due to its anticlotting action and is listed in most state protocols following the American Heart Association™ guidelines. Aspirin is also indicated for headache and other pain, but not usually in the emergency setting.

145. C

The police may obtain a copy of the report if they either get permission from the patient or obtain a search warrant from a judge or magistrate. Note the use of the qualifying word *routinely* in the question.

146. D

As already stated, improper restraint technique can lead to apnea and sudden death. If correct protocols are not followed, then the EMT may be open to criminal charges of assault and battery, false imprisonment, and kidnapping. A violent patient is at risk for injury, as are the EMTs who have responded. Improperly applied restraints can cause injury to the patient or the EMTs if the patient manages to extricate him or herself.

147. A

A first pregnancy will normally have a longer labor and delivery time than the subsequent pregnancies.

148. B

The ambulance should be used to protect the scene in order to avoid injury to the EMTs and the patients.

149. B

The second stage of labor occurs when the baby is forced out of the uterus by the contractions down into the mother's vagina and ends with the birth of the baby. The first stage of labor is from the expulsion of the mucous plug through the baby's expulsion from the uterus, and the third stage follows the birth of the baby when the placenta is delivered. There is no fourth stage of labor.

150. C

Implied consent means that in the case of a patient who cannot give consent, such as an individual who is unconscious, consent for treatment is implied and constitutes what the average person would want under similar circumstances.

YOUR PRACTICE TEST SCORES

The Practice Test in this book is designed to provide practice answering EMT-Basic-style questions along with a review of EMT-Basic content. Your results on this test indicate where you are NOW. It is not designed to predict your ability to pass the EMT-Basic exam.

- If you scored 70 percent or better, you have a good understanding of essential EMT-Basic content and are able to use the knowledge and thinking skills required to answer exam-style questions.

- If you scored 60 to 69 percent, you have areas of EMT-Basic content that need further review, and/or you may need continued work to master the knowledge and thinking skills required to be successful on the EMT-Basic exam.

- If you scored 59 percent or less, you need concentrated study of EMT-Basic content and continued practice utilizing the knowledge and thinking skills required to be successful on the EMT-Basic exam.

If you need more review, use the bulleted lists at the beginning of each chapter to find the subjects you need more practice on. Do the review questions at the end of each chapter and read the answer explanations to reinforce your learning. Take a look at the test-taking strategies and read "Test Mentality" in chapter one, then relax! You're ready, and you're going to do a great job.

EMT-Basic Resources

Glossary

Abandonment. The failure to properly treat an ill or injured person who is in need of emergency medical care.

Abdominal quadrants. The four sections of the abdomen, as defined by using the umbilicus, or navel, as the focal point: upper left, upper right, lower left, lower right.

Abrasion. A type of wound in which the dermis is scraped by an object, causing little blood loss but with increased danger of infection due to the amount of epidermis exposed.

Activated charcoal. Charcoal in liquid suspension used to absorb ingested poisons.

Active rewarming. Use of heat packs and heated fluids to rewarm a hypothermic patient.

Acute. Immediate.

Adolescent. Pediatric patient between 12 and 18 years of age.

Advance directive. Medical decisions made by a patient or caregiver in advance, usually in the form of do-not-resuscitate orders.

Afterbirth. The expulsion of the placenta from the mother following delivery of a baby.

Allergic reaction. The severe and unusual response of the body to a foreign substance.

Altered mental status. An inappropriate response to normal stimuli, such as responsive only to voice, responsive only to pain, or unconscious; also used to describe aberrant behavior.

Alveoli. Sacs in the lung in which oxygen is exchanged for carbon dioxide in the red blood cells.

Amniotic sac. The bag of fluid that surrounds and protects the fetus during pregnancy. This bag usually ruptures prior to delivery.

Amputation. The complete separation of a body part from the body.

Anaphylaxis. The consequence of an allergic reaction, in which the body responds with swelling of respiratory tissues and shock.

Aorta. Large artery at the top of the heart carrying blood to all of the major arteries.

Apnea. Lack of breathing, absence of respiratory activity.

Arterioles. Small arteries that connect the arteries to the capillaries.

Arteriosclerosis. Disease process in which the arteries lose elasticity as they become rigid; also known as hardening of the arteries.

Arteries. Vessel that carry oxygenated blood from the aorta to the arterioles.

Aspiration. Inhaling of foreign substances into the trachea, bronchial tree, and lungs.

Asystole. Cardiac standstill, lack of electrical activity in the heart muscle.

Atria. The two uppermost chambers of the heart.

Aura. Visual, auditory, olfactory, or other sense of an impending seizure.

Auscultation. Listening for sounds within the body, usually with a stethoscope.

Automated External Defibrillator (AED). A device that attempts to overcome certain cardiac dysrhythmias with an electrical countershock and operates by interpreting the cardiac rhythm and responding appropriately without the need for operator interpretation.

AVPU. Acronym used for determining level of consciousness: Alert, responsive to Verbal, responsive to Pain, Unresponsive.

Avulsion. Forcible tearing away of tissue as a result of blunt-force trauma.

Bag-Valve Mask. Respiratory device used to manually support respirations in a patient in respiratory distress or apnea.

Bandage. Cloth used to secure a sterile dressing to a wound.

Baseline vital signs. Vital signs taken first and used to track a patient's improvement or decline.

Battle's Sign. Ecchymosis behind the ears that suggests a basilar skull fracture.

Behavioral emergency. An emergency medical call in which the patient's actions are bizarre and inappropriate.

Bilateral. Referring to both the right and left sides of the body.

Bipolar disorder. Psychiatric condition in which a patient alternates between extremes of euphoria and depression. These extremes may last from a few minutes to several months.

Blood pressure. The pressure in millimeters of mercury of the blood flow through the arteries.

Body substance isolation (BSI). The important act of protection of an EMT from airborne and bloodborne pathogens by the use of personal protective equipment (PPE).

Brachial artery. The large artery in the upper arm that feeds the entire extremity.

Bradycardia. Heart rate slower than 60 beats per minute.

Bradypnea. Respiratory rate slower than eight respirations per minute.

Breech birth. Presentation of any part of a fetus other than the head during delivery.

Bronchi. Two tubes that connect the trachea to the bronchioles.

Bronchioles. Smaller tubes that connect the bronchi to the alveoli.

Burn sheet. Large sterile dressing used to cover burn injuries.

Capillaries. Small blood vessels in which oxygen is given off to the cells for metabolism and waste products are collected.

Capillary refill. Diagnostic sign in which the nail bed is blanched by applying pressure and the time for it to return to normal color is measured, normally less than two seconds.

Cardiac arrest. Condition caused by the heart's failure to pump blood.

Carotid arteries. Large arteries that feed the brain.

Central nervous system (CNS). The brain and spinal cord.

Cerebrovascular accident. Ischemia in the brain caused by either a cerebral hemorrhage or thrombus; also known as a stroke.

Chief complaint. Illness or injury for which the emergency medical system was activated.

Chronic obstructive pulmonary disease (COPD). Degeneration of the alveoli by disease processes causing progressive dyspnea; examples are emphysema and chronic bronchitis.

Chronic. Long-term gradual process.

Conduction. Method of heat transfer in which heat is transferred by direct contact between bodies.

Congestive heart failure (CHF). Condition of dyspnea in which fluid backs up into the lungs caused by failure of the heart's pumping action.

Contraindications. Situations in which a drug or protocol should not be used.

Contusion. Hemorrhage that occurs beneath the skin; bruising.

Convection. Method of heat transfer from the body caused by air passing over it.

Convulsion. Seizure activity of the body.

Critical incident stress debriefing (CISD). Discussion of a stressful incident, with the goal of allowing an EMT to deal with the emotions encountered and move on.

Crowning. The appearance of the top of the baby's head in the birth canal during delivery.

Cushing's reflex. Increased blood pressure, decreased heart rate, and respiratory changes caused by hypoxia in the brain; indicative of severe head injury.

Cyanosis. Bluish-gray color indicative of poor circulatory perfusion.

Decerebrate posturing. When a patient extends arms outward and arches the back; an indication of severe head injury.

Decorticate posturing. When a patient flexes arms inward and arches the back; an indication of a more severe head injury.

Defibrillation. Correction of cardiac fibrillation by electrical countershock.

Dementia. Abnormal behavior brought about by disease of the brain.

Dermis. Intermediate layer of skin between the epidermis and fatty tissue or muscle.

Diabetes. Disease of the pancreas that inhibits the body's ability to process sugars.

Diastolic blood pressure. Pressure in the arteries while the heart is at rest.

Dressing. Sterile pad placed directly on a wound.

Drowning. Death caused by suffocation in water.

Drug. Any chemical introduced into the body to combat disease.

Dyspnea. Difficulty breathing.

Ecchymosis. Black-and-blue discoloration caused by subcutaneous hemorrhage.

Endocrine system. System of the body that produces hormones used in the metabolic process.

Epidermis. Top layer of skin.

Epidural. Layer between the skull and the dural matter of the brain and spine.

Epilepsy. Disease of the brain that causes seizures. Also known as seizure disorder.

Epinephrine. Natural hormone that helps the body regulate multiple processes. Also a medication used for various heart irregularities and anaphylaxis.

Epistaxis. Bleeding from the nose.

Esophagus. The body's tubular passage from the pharynx to the stomach.

Evisceration. Traumatic opening of the abdominal cavity in which the intestines protrude to the outside.

Expressed consent. Formal consent from a competent patient for treatment and/or transport.

Extubation. Removal of a breathing tube.

Femoral artery. Large artery in the upper leg that feeds the entire extremity.

Femur. Large bone of the upper leg.

Fetus. Child in the uterus before birth.

Fibula. One of two bones in the lower leg.

Flail segment. Two or more ribs broken in two or more places.

Fontanel. Soft spot in a baby's skull where the bones have not yet grown together.

Fowler's position. Position of a patient in which the patient is sitting upright. This is normally the best position for conscious patients with dyspnea.

French catheter. Soft-suction catheter.

Full-thickness burn. Burn that extends through the epidermis and dermis to the tissues below. Formally known as a third-degree burn.

Glucose. Form of sugar used by the body for fuel.

Guarding. Position in which a patient places his or her hands over a portion of the anatomy that is painful.

Hard catheter. Rigid-suction catheter.

Hazardous material. Any material that is dangerous to one's health or safety.

Head-tilt chin-lift. Procedure of securing the airway of a nontrauma patient by placing one hand on the patient's forehead and tilting it back while simultaneously lifting the chin with the other hand.

Hives. Itchy, red blotches on the skin associated with allergic reactions.

Hot zone. In a hazardous-materials incident, the area that contains the hazardous material causing the incident. Only personnel in proper protective equipment for the hazard should enter this zone.

Hyper-. Prefix denoting higher, more, faster.

Hyperthermia. Overheated, having a high temperature

Hypo-. Prefix denoting lower, below, less, slower.

Hypoglycemia. Low blood sugar.

Hypothermia. Cold, having a low temperature.

Hypovolemia. Low blood volume.

Hypoxia. Low oxygen level.

Immune response. Body's response to a foreign invader.

Implied consent. Assumption that consent would be given for treatment or transport if the patient were conscious.

Incident command system. System of command and control at a mass casualty or disaster scene.

Indications. Situations in which a drug or protocol should be followed.

Infant. Pediatric patient between the ages of 1 month and 12 months.

Ingestion. Process in which an object is taken into the mouth and swallowed.

Inhalation. Process in which an object is brought into the lungs through the nose and mouth. Also known as inspiration.

Initial assessment. First impression of a patient's condition after scene size-up.

Injection. Process in which a substance is introduced into the body by a needle.

In-line stabilization. Holding of the head and neck in a straight-line neutral position to minimize danger of damaging the spinal cord during treatment and transport.

Insulin. Hormone used by the body to metabolize sugars.

Intercostal muscles. Muscles between the ribs used in the breathing process.

Intracranial pressure (ICP). Pressure within the skull.

Intubation. Act of placing a tube into the trachea to facilitate rescue breathing.

Jaundice. Yellowish appearance of the skin, commonly caused by diseases of the liver.

Jaw-thrust maneuver. Maneuver to open the airway of a trauma patient. Head and neck are maintained in a neutral position, and the jaw is lifted upward to open the airway.

Joint. Location in which two bones meet.

Kinetics. Study of physical laws of motion (used for trauma assessment).

Labor. Process through which a baby is born. Labor begins when the mucus plug blocking the cervix is expelled and concludes with the delivery of the placenta.

Laceration. Wound in which the skin is opened by a cut or tear.

Ligaments. Bands of tissue that connect muscles, bones, and joints.

Lungs. Organs comprised of small air sacs in which oxygenated air is inhaled and passes into the blood and carbon-dioxide waste is removed.

Main stem bronchi. Large tubes connecting the trachea to the lungs.

Malaise. General feeling of illness.

Mammalian diving reflex. Body's response to sudden immersion into cold water in which vital systems shut down to preserve oxygen.

Mantoux test. Test for tuberculosis bacteria.

Mechanism of injury (MOI). The manner in which an injury occurs.

Meconium. Waste product expelled by a distressed fetus during delivery.

Medical control. The EMT's supervising medical professional(s).

Medical direction. Protocols and practices given to EMTs by a physician.

Medication. Any substance introduced into a body to affect healing or alleviation of abnormal symptoms.

Meninges. Layers of tissue surrounding the brain and spinal cord.

Metered dose inhaler. Device prescribed to patients to deliver a prescribed dosage of medication to be inhaled. Usually prescribed for asthma and other respiratory illnesses.

Minor consent. Permission obtained from a responsible adult for a minor child or incapacitated adult.

Miscarriage. Expulsion of a fetus and products of conception before the fetus is viable.

Multiple casualty incident (MCI). An incident with one or more patients than the initial arriving unit can safely treat and transport.

KAPLAN

Nasal cannula. Oxygen delivery device that delivers two to six liters per minute into the nasopharynx.

Nasogastric tube. Tube inserted into the nose and down into the stomach to suction possible toxins and/or administer medication directly into the stomach.

Nasopharyngeal airway. An airway device inserted into the nose and nasopharynx.

Nature of illness (NOI). Signs and symptoms of patient's illness.

Negligence. Legally defined as failure to act as a reasonable and prudent person would under similar circumstances.

Neonate. Pediatric patient from birth to one month old.

Nervous system. System of sensory and motor nerves that control the human body functions, both voluntary and involuntary.

Neurogenic shock. A type of shock brought about by damage to the central nervous system that causes vasodilation and resulting hypovolemia.

Neurological deficit. Any lessening or absence of the body's nervous-system response.

Nitroglycerin (NTG). Medication used for chest pain that causes vasodilation, which increases oxygen flow to the heart.

Nonrebreather mask. Oxygen delivery device that delivers 10–15 liters per minute; the reservoir bag provides 100 percent oxygen to the patient.

Obstetric. Having to do with delivery or childbirth.

Occlusive dressing. Sterile covering that seals off the wound from air; dressings of impermeable material or impregnated with sterile petroleum jelly.

Offline medical direction. Written standard protocols from an EMS medical director.

Ongoing assessment. The continuous monitoring of a patient while en route to a receiving facility.

Online medical direction. Direct contact with a physician to obtain orders or consultation.

Open fracture. A broken bone associated with an open wound.

Oral airway. A device that assists in holding the tongue clear of the airway and maintaining a clear passage through the oropharynx.

Oral glucose. High concentration of sugar given orally to a conscious patient in hypoglycemia.

Orbits. The openings in the skull for the eyeballs.

Oropharyngeal airway. A specific type of oral airway, shaped like the letter J and inserted into the mouth to hold the tongue down.

Overdose. Misuse of any substance by ingesting, inhaling, or absorbing more than needed.

Oxygen humidifier. Bottle of sterile water placed in-line with oxygen flow to provide moisture and prevent drying out of the pharynx.

Oxygen. Element used by the body for metabolism, constituting 20 percent of normal air. Supplemental oxygen is often given to assist breathing and metabolism in times of illness or injury.

Pallor. Pale or abnormally light skin color.

Palpation. Feeling with the hands and fingers.

Paradoxical motion. Opposite motion from the norm. Used to describe the effect when a flail segment moves in an opposite-to-normal direction during breathing.

Paranoia. Mental illness categorized by deep feelings of persecution.

Paresthesia. Loss of sensation or paralysis in an extremity.

Partial-thickness burn. Burn that extends through the epidermis and dermis but not below causing blistering. Formally known as a second-degree burn.

Passive rewarming. Reheating of a hypothermic patient by raising the ambient temperature, removing cold and wet clothing, and applying blankets to utilize the patient's own body heat.

Patent airway. Open, secure airway.

Pathogens. Substances that cause disease.

Patient assessment. Medical examination to determine mechanisms of injury and manner of illnesses.

Perfusion. Physiology of delivery of oxygen to the cells for the metabolic process.

Peritonitis. Infection of the abdominal cavity.

Personal protective equipment. Any device used by an EMT to protect against airborne and bloodborne pathogens.

Pharynx. Area between the mouth and the epiglottis, in which the trachea and esophagus separate.

Phobia. Mental illness manifesting itself in irrational fears.

Physiology. Study of the body's systems and functions.

Placenta. Organ that feeds the fetus during pregnancy. It attaches to the wall of the uterus and is discharged following delivery of the fetus.

Plasma. Liquid component of blood.

Platelets. Component of blood that produces the clotting effect.

Pleural space. Space between the outer walls of the lungs.

Pneumothorax. Collapse of the lung caused by air build-up in the chest.

Pocket mask. Device for providing artificial ventilation by allowing an EMT to utilize his own exhalation to inflate a victim's lungs.

Poison. Any substance that inhibits the body's normal processes.

Positive pressure ventilation. Method of ventilation in which the lungs are inflated by a device that forces air in; may be a mechanical ventilator, pocket mask, or a bag-valve mask.

Postictal state. State of unconsciousness following a seizure.

Prehospital care report (PCR). Summary of observations and interactions between the emergency medical service and a patient. The PCR is left with the receiving facility to become a permanent part of the patient's record.

Premature infant. Infant who is delivered before 36 weeks of gestation.

Preschooler. Pediatric patient between the ages of three and six years of age.

Pressure point. Place in which an artery crosses a bone and pressure can reduce hemorrhage.

Primary triage. In an MCI, the first categorization of degree of injury, with the primary goal of identifying the most severely injured patients and prioritizing them for treatment and transport.

Prolapsed cord. Abnormal delivery situation in which the umbilical cord presents from the birth canal before the fetus.

Prone. Position of a body facedown.

Protocols. Series of directives approved by a medical director for EMS to follow in given situations.

Pulmonary edema. Fluid in the lungs.

Pulmonary embolism. Blockage in the circulatory system of the lungs.

Pulse oximetry. Measurement of oxygen perfusion, measured by the infrared signature of red blood cells.

Pulse pressure. Difference between the systolic and diastolic blood pressure.

Pulseless electrical activity (PEA). Random electrical activity of the heart that fails to produce a pulse.

Pulse. Movement of blood through the arteries caused by contraction of the left ventricle.

Raccoon sign. Ecchymosis around the eyes, which may be symptomatic of a basilar skull fracture.

Radiation. Method of heat transfer in which there is no direct contact between bodies.

Rapid extrication. Method of removal of a patient from a hazardous situation without using normal precautions due to imminent danger.

Rapid medical assessment. Method of assessing an unconscious patient from head to toe to ascertain medical problems and to check for injuries.

Rapid trauma assessment. Method of assessing an unconscious patient from head to toe to check for injuries if there is a substantial mechanism of injury.

Reasonable force. Legal definition used to describe the minimum amount of force needed to restrain a patient in order to prevent injury to the patient or others.

Red blood cells. Component of the blood that carries oxygen to the cells.

Repeaters. Radios that amplify a radio signal and enable it to carry longer distances.

Respiration. Inhaling oxygen into the lungs for the metabolic process.

Respiratory arrest. Absence of spontaneous respirations.

Respiratory failure. Inability of the body to bring in adequate oxygen for the metabolic process.

Retractions. Depressions in the neck and chest cavity indicating use of the accessory muscles for respirations; indicative of respiratory distress.

Right main stem intubation. Placing of an endotracheal tube too far into the trachea and into the right main stem bronchus, resulting in the inflation of only the right lung.

Rigid catheter. Hard plastic suction device; also known as a tonsil-tip suction.

Route. Manner of drug delivery, i.e., oral, intravenous, etc.

Rule of nines. Method of dividing an adult body into 11 zones of nine percent each to rapidly determine how extensive a burn injury is.

SAMPLE. Diagnostic mnemonic that stands for: **S**igns and **S**ymptoms, **A**llergies, **M**edications, **P**ertinent history, **L**ast oral intake, and **E**vents leading to current illness or injury.

Scene safety. Primary concern of an arriving EMT that the situation in which he or she is arriving is as hazard-free as possible.

Scene size-up. Quick assessment of a scene upon arrival to determine scene safety, number of victims and need for additional or special units.

Schizophrenia. Mental illness categorized by delusions, blunted affect, thought disorders, and sometimes catatonia.

School age. Pediatric patient between the ages of 6 and 12 years of age.

Scope of practice. Medical procedures that are legally permitted to any individual dependent on level of licensure and training.

Secondary triage. In an MCI, triage of a specific patient's condition to determine treatment and transport.

Seizure. Involuntary muscle tremors or loss of consciousness.

Semi-Fowler position. Position of a patient in which the patient is sitting at a 45-degree angle. This is normally the best position for conscious patients with mild dyspnea and cardiac symptoms.

Shock. Situation in which cells are not properly oxygenated due to loss of blood, also known as hypoperfusion syndrome.

Side effects. Effects of any drug or procedure other than its intended effect.

Signs. Objective measurements of a body's response to illness and/or injury.

Snoring. Sound made by a partial obstruction of the upper airway.

Soft catheter. Suction device of soft plastic; also called a French catheter.

Sphygmomanometer. Device used to measure blood pressure by applying pressure to an artery; also known as a blood pressure cuff.

Spinal column. Bony structure of the back that protects the spinal cord.

Spinal cord. Series of nerves leading from the base of the brain that carry impulses to the muscles and sensory information back to the brain.

Spinal shock. Shock caused by injury to the spinal cord that affects its ability to transmit the necessary nerve impulses for normal perfusion.

Splint. Any device that immobilizes a bone or joint.

Spontaneous abortion. Any termination of pregnancy that occurs before a fetus is able to remain viable; also known as miscarriage.

Staging sector. Section where units are deployed to remain ready to respond to specific assignments at a mass casualty incident.

Standard of care. Level of medical treatment that is normal and expected for a given situation.

Standing orders. Procedures that medical control deems suitable for the EMT to perform under given situations without the need to contract medical control. (See **offline medical direction**.)

Status epilepticus. Seizures that last longer than a few minutes or multiple seizures that occur without an intervening period of lucidity.

Sterile. Objects free from pathogens.

Stoma. Opening in the neck bypassing the pharynx to enable breathing.

Stridor. High-pitched wheezing sound indicating upper airway swelling or obstruction.

Stroke. Brain damage caused by a clot or hemorrhage in the cerebrum or cerebellum. Also known as a cerebral vascular accident, or CVA.

Stylet. Semirigid rod used to shape an endotracheal tube for insertion.

Subarachnoid hemorrhage. Bleeding between the brain and the arachnoid membrane.

Subcutaneous layer. Layer of tissue directly below the skin.

Subdural hematoma. Bleeding beneath the dura, or outer covering of the brain.

Sucking chest wound. Open wound that extends into the lung cavity, causing deflation of the lung (pneumothorax).

Sudden infant death syndrome (SIDS). Medical condition affecting infants who die suddenly and without any explanation.

Suicide. The taking of one's own life.

Superficial burn. A burn that involves only the epidermis. Formerly known as a first-degree burn. A common sunburn is an example of a superficial burn.

Supine hypotensive syndrome. Condition which occurs in late pregnancy in which the weight of the fetus impairs the return circulation of blood and causes low blood pressure and inadequate perfusion.

Supply sector. MCI location where supplies are brought for units to restock.

Symptoms. Subjective description of various processes by a patient.

Syncope. Brief period of loss of consciousness.

Systolic blood pressure. Pressure in the arteries while the ventricles contract.

Tachycardia. Sustained fast heart rate in excess of 100 beats per minute.

Tachypnea. Sustained fast respiratory rate in excess of 20 breaths per minute.

Tension pneumothorax. Condition caused by the collapse of a lung in which the organs in the chest begin to shift into the space vacated by the collapsed lung.

Tidal volume. The amount of air inhaled in a normal respiratory effort.

Toddler. Pediatric patient between the ages of 1 and 3 years.

Toxin. Substance that poisons the body.

Trachea. Tube connecting the mouth and nose to the lungs.

Tracheostomy. Surgical opening in the neck enabling a patient with an occluded airway to breathe.

Transient ischemic attack (TIA). Medical condition that causes temporary strokelike symptoms, caused by spasms of the arteries in the brain.

Transportation sector. In an MCI, the area in which patients are transported to appropriate medical facilities.

Trauma. Sudden injury caused by the application of external forces to a human body.

Treatment sector. In an MCI, the area in which patients are given initial treatment before transport.

Trendelenburg position. Supine positioning of the body with legs elevated in order to combat shock.

Triage. The process of determining the severity of injuries in order to best utilize available resources. The triage process normally has four groups: red for critical patients, yellow for serious patients, green for slightly injured ambulatory patients, and black for patients who are dead or mortally wounded.

Triage sector. In an MCI, the area in which triage occurs and is controlled. Initial triage occurs where the patient is found.

Triage tag. A tag that enables the EMT to mark the patient's status and initial impressions. It is also used to account for patients as they pass through the various sectors.

Tripod position. Position that a patient in severe respiratory distress often assumes, seated with arms to the side and rotated forward to facilitate breathing.

Umbilical cord. Vessel that connects a fetus to the placenta in utero.

Umbilicus. The navel; the area where the umbilical cord is connected to a fetus's abdomen.

Urgent move. Situation in which a patient is moved quickly due to either the seriousness of his or her condition or immediate danger of further injury.

Uterus. Female organ that harbors a fetus during pregnancy.

Vein. Blood vessel that carries blood toward the heart.

Venae cavae. Main veins leading directly into the heart.

Ventilation. Passage of air into and out of the lungs.

Ventricles. The two lower chambers of the heart.

Ventricular fibrillation (V-Fib). Cardiac condition in which the heart muscles vibrate rather than contract, resulting in collapse of circulation.

Ventricular tachycardia (V-Tach). Rapid heartbeat that frequently fails to produce a pulse and thus fails to produce perfusion.

Venules. Small blood vessels leading from the capillaries to the veins.

Vital signs. Assessments of an ill or injured patient that are objectively measured, including blood pressure, heart rate, respiratory rate, pupil response, and oxygen saturation.

Voluntary guarding. Contractions of the abdominal wall as a response to pain or injury.

Warm zone. In a hazardous-material incident, the area adjacent to the hot zone that injured patients are removed to for decontamination, triage, and treatment.

Water chill. Increase in loss of body heat due to presence of water.

White blood cells. Component of the blood that combats infection in the body.

Wind chill. Increase in loss of body heat due to wind speed.

Withdrawal. Body's response to the cessation of use of alcohol or narcotic substances.

Xiphoid process. Bony inferior tip of the sternum.

State EMS Certification Links

Alabama

Emergency Medical Services Division

http://www.adph.org/ems

Alaska

Emergency Medical Services

http://www.chems.alaska.gov/EMS/default.htm

Arizona

Bureau of Emergency Medical Services

http://www.azdhs.gov/bems

Arkansas

Emergency Medical Services and Trauma Systems

http://www.healthyarkansas.com/ems

California

Emergency Medical Services Authority

http://www.emsa.ca.gov

Colorado

Emergency Medical and Trauma Services

http://www.cdphe.state.co.us/em/emhom.html

Connecticut

Emergency Medical Services

http://www.dph.state.ct.us/OHCPHHO/EMS_Office/pages/education_main.htm

District of Columbia

Fire and Emergency Medical Services

http://fems.dc.gov/fems/site/default.asp

Delaware

Emergency Medical Services

http://www.state.de.us/dhss/dph/ems/ems.html

Florida

Bureau of Emergency Medical Services

http://www.doh.state.fl.us/ems

Georgia

Emergency Medical Services

http://health.state.ga.us/programs/ems/index.asp

Hawaii

Emergency Medical Services Program

http://www.chems.alaska.gov/EMS/default.htm

Idaho

Emergency Medical Services

http://www.healthandwelfare.idaho.gov/portal/alias__Rainbow/lang__en-US/tabID__3344/DesktopDefault.aspx

Illinois

Emergency Medical Services

http://www.ilems.com

Indiana

Emergency Medical Services

http://www.state.in.us/sema/ems

Iowa

Bureau of Emergency Medical Services

http://www.idph.state.ia.us/ems/default.asp

Kansas

Board of Emergency Medical Services

http://www.ksbems.org

Kentucky

Board of Emergency Medical Services

http://kbems.ky.gov

Louisiana

Emergency Medical Services

http://www.oph.dhh.state.la.us/emergencymedical/index.html

Maine

Maine Emergency Medical Services

http://www.state.me.us/dps/ems

Maryland

Institute for Emergency Medical Services Systems

http://miemss.umaryland.edu

Massachusetts

Office of Emergency Medical Services

http://www.mass.gov/dph/oems/oems.htm

Michigan

Emergency Medical Services

http://www.michigan.gov/mdch/0,1607,7-132-27417_27529_27537—-,00.html

Michigan

Dept. Of Community Health

http://www.michigan.gov/mdch

Minnesota

Emergency Medical Services Regulatory Board

http://www.emsrb.state.mn.us

Mississippi

Emergency Medical Services

http://www.ems.doh.ms.gov/ems/index.html

Missouri

Emergency Medical Services

http://www.health.state.mo.us/EMS

Montana

EMS & Trauma Systems

http://www.dphhs.state.mt.us/hpsd/pubheal/healsafe/ems/index.htm

Nebraska

Emergency Medical Services

http://www.hhs.state.ne.us/ems/emsindex.htm

Nevada

Emergency Medical Services

http://health2k.state.nv.us/ems/index.htm

New Hampshire

Bureau of Emergency Medical Services

http://www.nh.gov/safety/ems

New Jersey

Office of Emergency Medical Services

http://www.state.nj.us/health/ems/index.html

New Mexico

Emergency Medical Services Bureau

http://www.ipems.org

New York

Bureau of Emergency Medical Services

http://www.health.state.ny.us/nysdoh/ems/main.htm

North Carolina

Office of Emergency Medical Services

http://facility-services.state.nc.us/EMS/ems.htm

North Dakota

Division of Emergency Medical Services

http://www.health.state.nd.us/ndhd/resource/dehs

Ohio

Division of Emergency Medical Services

http://www.ems.ohio.gov

Oklahoma

Emergency Medical Services Division

http://www.health.state.ok.us/program/ems/index.html

Oregon

Emergency Medical Services and Trauma Systems

http://www.ohd.hr.state.or.us/ems/index.cfm

Pennsylvania

Emergency Medical Services

http://www.dsf.health.state.pa.us/health/cwp/view.asp?a=170&Q=203353

South Carolina

Emergency Medical Services

http://www.scdhec.net/hr/ems

South Dakota

Office of Emergency Medical Services

http://www.state.sd.us/dps/ems/index.htm

Tennessee

Emergency Medical Services

http://www2.state.tn.us/health/ems

Texas

Emergency Medical Services

http://www.tdh.state.tx.us/hcqs/ems/default.htm

Utah

Bureau of Emergency Medical Services

http://health.utah.gov/ems

Vermont

Emergency Medical Services

http://www.healthyvermonters.info/hp/ems/emshome.shtml

Virginia

Office of Emergency Medical Services

http://www.vdh.state.va.us/oems

Washington

Office of Emergency and Trauma Prevention

http://www.doh.wa.gov/hsqa/emtp

West Virginia

Office of Emergency Medical Services

http://www.wvoems.org

Wisconsin

Emergency Medical Services

http://dhfs.wisconsin.gov/ems

Wyoming

Emergency Medical Services

http://wdhfs.state.wy.us/ems/abama